AF582894

The Best Of All Things

A Tapestry of Faith, Hope, Resilience, and the Human Connection

Rejoice always, pray continually, give thanks in all circumstances; for this is God's will for you in Christ Jesus.

1 Thessalonians 5: 16-18 NIV

Dr. Sómone D. Washington

ISBN: 979-8-218-49991-4

This book is based on true events. Some names and identifying details have been changed to protect the privacy of individuals.

For those who are currently on dialysis, waiting patiently for their second chance at life.

Foreword

When Ms. Washington asked me to do the Forward for this book, I was very excited. I felt honored as I read and RE-read her book about her dialysis and transplant journey! This book brought back memories of my own time on dialysis which, between 1972 and 1975, weren't the most pleasant things for me to remember. However, as with all things there were happy times and laughter.

I was one of five kids undergoing dialysis together, and we had the absolute best dialysis technicians and nurses on the planet. They did their best to distract us from those very loud machines that were taking our blood away, cleansing it and sending it back to us in those plastic tubes, but I more easily remember the exploding coils, the legs cramps, and pain of my dialysis days.

Unlike today, the cell phone days, we carried beepers to receive communication from the Transplant Center requesting us come into the Center to get tissue typed for a possible kidney. It happened to me several times as it happened to Ms. Washington, with that final contact being the best news ever for both of us! There was finally an available kidney.

While my library contains over a dozen books written by transplant recipients, from short stories about times in "the John" to a true-life story about Maggot Therapy, THIS is the book that I believe takes us on the dialysis and transplant journey in a most interesting way! A journey full of ups and downs, twists and turns! This is a true-life story that you will read and re-read, and it can actually help direct you on your own organ transplant journey.

As her life has gotten back to a more normal state because of her transplant, my hope and I'm sure her hope is that all who need a transplant will get one. Sadly, unless we work to get the word out about the true need of more organs, many of those needing one will die waiting. That's the reality we all face.

Continue to get that word out folks!

George E. Franklin, III
Longest Surviving African-American Deceased Donor Kidney Recipient (49 years to date)

Preface

I believe in the transformative power of open dialogue. No topic is too sensitive, no question too bold. Through honest conversations, we forge connections that lead to deeper understanding and clarity, helping us refine our personal values and beliefs. These exchanges not only provide a platform for self-expression but also cultivate the courage to articulate our thoughts and feelings. At their best, such conversations bring healing to the heart, mind, and spirit, allowing relationships to flourish, mend, and deepen.

This philosophy is why I embrace the question, "What happened to your arm?" regardless of who asks or when. I welcome this inquiry as an opportunity to share my journey through diagnosis, dialysis, and kidney transplantation—a journey that resonates with many who have faced similar health challenges, either personally or through loved ones. Each interaction, however brief, leaves a mark on my life and contributes to the vital conversation surrounding organ, eye, and tissue donation.

Over the past 13 years, these dialogues have often led to the suggestion, "You should write a book." Following the passing of my beloved father, Henry Washington, in September 2022, I finally found the encouragement I needed to embark on this writing journey. What began as journal entries has evolved into the narrative you are about to explore.

This book aims to restore hope to those undergoing dialysis and offer practical advice for family and friends on how to tangibly support loved ones living with chronic illness. It sheds light on how the selfless decisions of donor families can profoundly impact lives and serve as a call to action for everyone to register as organ, eye, and tissue donors.

As you delve into these pages, I invite you to discover yourself within the stories and insights shared. May you emerge with a renewed perspective on what it means to leave a lasting legacy.

Contents

I know what it is to be in need, and I know what it is to have plenty. I have learned the secret of being content in any and every situation, whether well fed or hungry, whether living in plenty or in want. I can do all this through Him who gives me strength.

–Philippians 4: 12-13

1.
From Miami to MegaFest

At twenty-four years old, I am healthy, vibrant, and full of life. My days are spent as a Computer Specialist at Biscayne Gardens Elementary School, where I maintain networks, software, and equipment, while contributing to the nurturing of young minds through technology. Evenings are reserved for my studies at Barry University, where I'm on the cusp of completing my Master of Science degree in Information Technology, set to graduate in December. I navigate my single life in North Miami, actively dating and enjoying the independence of my own apartment.

My journey into sorority sisterhood began four years prior and on April 1, 2000, I crossed into Delta Sigma Theta Sorority, Inc., Iota Pi Citywide Chapter at Florida International University. Earning my Bachelor's degree in Business Administration with a major in Management Information Systems was a pivotal moment, and my five sorority line sisters and I continue to share laughter and camaraderie, experiencing life together. While things may not be perfect, I embrace my life as it is — a beautiful tapestry woven with moments and memories.

For the past three years, I have been a member of Antioch Missionary Baptist Church of Miami Gardens, where Pastor Arthur Jackson, III leads the congregation. Though the church is vibrant and thriving, its size sometimes leaves me feeling disconnected. In my quest for deeper spiritual growth, I seek connections beyond the Sunday service.

Fortunately, I work alongside incredible women of faith who are true prayer warriors. My immediate supervisor, Mrs. Gardenia Bulluck, the Instructional Technology Specialist, along with her colleagues and friends Dr. Beverly Corridon, the Science Coach, and the Mathematics Coach, share a unique bond. Every morning, they gather in their adjoining offices, sipping coffee and engaging in worship while the local news softly plays from the television in the background.

One day, eager to get a jump on my work, I arrived early and stumbled into their morning gathering. Their invitation for me to join them felt like divine intervention. I quickly became part of their circle, absorbing their insights and learning the art of purposeful prayer. Our mornings together transformed into deep friendships, one of which later included Marjorie Banks, a newer addition to the fold who further enriched our group. I was starting to realize that I was surrounded by truly powerful women of God.

”

I found the spiritual daily bread that I was looking for, learning how to articulate purposeful prayers, and absorbing the wisdom of the intelligent and God-fearing women around me.

As our morning devotions deepened our bond, an exciting opportunity arose—a road trip to the inaugural Gospel MegaFest Conference in Atlanta, Georgia, hosted by Bishop TD Jakes. Though my finances were tight, having just given my last dollars as an offering at church, Dr. Corridon and Marjorie encouraged me to step out in faith, trusting that God would provide a way for me to attend. With their encouragement, I took the leap.

On Thursday, Banks, Dr. Corridon, and I arrived at MegaFest, and my heart raced as I approached the ticket window, debit card in hand. I prayed silently, hoping the transaction would go through. To my amazement, it did. I had forgotten that direct deposit employees receive their paychecks a day early, a blessing I had unknowingly been granted.

The speakers at MegaFest delivered messages that resonated deeply within me, and I left feeling spiritually charged and ready to serve. My journey was not just about the destination; it was about the connections, the faith, and the unwavering belief that God's provision would always see me through. Life was unfolding beautifully, and I was ready to embrace every moment.

And my God will meet all your needs according to the riches of his glory in Christ Jesus.

-Philippians 4:19

Let's Chat About It:
From Miami to MegaFest

1. How did my experiences at 24 years old resonate with your own life experiences at that age?

2. In what ways did I find community and support among my colleagues? How does this reflect the importance of friendships in times of spiritual growth?

3. I took a leap of faith in attending the Gospel MegaFest despite financial concerns. Can you share a time when you stepped out in faith? What was the outcome?

4. The morning gatherings became a source of spiritual nourishment for me. How do you cultivate your own spiritual growth in your life?

5. I emphasize the bond formed with my sorority line sisters and prayer warriors. What role does sisterhood (or community) play in your life, and how has it impacted your personal journey?

6. What practical steps can we take to find and create supportive communities in our own lives, similar to my experience?

Share your thoughts by leaving a book review on Amazon.com. I would love to read it.

2.
A Journey to Jamaica

In July, Dr. Corridon and I received an invitation to The Faith Center, where a special guest pastor, Paula White, was scheduled to speak. I had never heard of her, but I thought, "Why not?" That evening, she delivered an inspiring message that resonated deeply with me. It turned out that she was a prominent pastor with her own television ministry on the Trinity Broadcasting Network (TBN), and soon after, TBN became a staple in my viewing routine.

At the end of the service, I met Jerelyn, the woman who had invited us. She shared her plans for a mission trip to Jamaica to deliver hurricane relief supplies following the devastation wrought by Hurricane Ivan. Jerelyn needed more people to join her to accommodate the donations on the plane, and after learning more about the mission, Dr. Corridon and I agreed to help.

With excitement, I applied for my first passport, which arrived just a month before our departure. Jerelyn invited us to join her in a 10-day Daniel Fast to bless our journey and honor God. I had never fasted before, nor had I ever traveled internationally, or even participated in a mission trip. But again, I thought, "Why not?"

The Daniel Fast is inspired by a biblical account found in the Book of Daniel, Chapter 1. When the king of Babylon sought to train young men from Jerusalem for service, including Daniel, he assigned them royal food and wine to eat and drink. Daniel, wishing to honor his culture and beliefs, requested to abstain from these provisions. Despite initial resistance, he persisted and was allowed to eat only vegetables and water, a decision that ultimately led to his favor.

> "Please test your servants for ten days: Give us nothing but vegetables to eat and water to drink. Then compare our appearance with that of the young men who ate the royal food and treat your servants in accordance with what you see." At the end of the ten days they looked healthier and better nourished than any of the young men who ate the royal food. To these four young men God gave knowledge and understanding of all kinds of literature and learning. And Daniel could understand visions and dreams of all kinds. At the end of the time set by the king to bring them into service... The king talked with them, and he found none equal to Daniel...; so they entered the king's service. In every matter of wisdom and understanding about which the king questioned them, he found them ten times better than all the magicians and enchanters in his whole kingdom.
> - Daniel 1:12-13, 15, 17-20 NIV

Because of the story of Daniel and his fast, many people still fast today as a means to gain discernment or clarity regarding a certain situation and/or a closer relationship with God.

During our fast, we consumed only fruit, vegetables, and water. The first two days were manageable, but by the third day, I struggled. Food cravings hit me hard, and hunger gnawed at my resolve. I occupied my mind with tasks, chugged water, and reminded myself of the greater purpose behind my sacrifice, which kept me from giving in. The seventh and ninth days echoed the third, but the others were easier to navigate.

Determined to deepen my connection with God during this fast, I followed Dr. Corridon's advice: I prayed, read Scripture, worshiped, and took moments of silence to listen for God's voice. Each day blended into a routine of early morning prayers, Bible reading, note-taking, TBN playing softly in the background, and listening to praise and worship music. The rhythm of prayer, reading, notes, TBN, worship, fruit, vegetables, water, and quiet time became my life.

Fasting Day 1 Journal Entry

Good morning, Lord. As You know, today is the first day of our fast. We are enduring Daniel's ten day fast as illustrated in Your Word in order to have clean bodies and clear minds for our mission in Jamaica later this month. I am excited to attempt this fast. This is something that I have never done before, but I understand it to be very important.

Your Word says that the men gained knowledge and understanding from You while fasting and because they fasted. That is very encouraging to me because like so many of Your children, there is so much that I would like to know. But I know that You will reveal what is necessary in Your own time.

I must tell You that my life changed so much when I really decided and put my mind to being your faithful servant. I know that the course of events that got me to this point was all from you and I know that I have been so stubborn and resistant in the past, but I'm finally here now, totally.

I'm not 100% sure exactly what that entails, but I am sure You will show me in Your own time.

I have to wholeheartedly thank You for all that You have shown me in the past two months. From showing me how far a sacrificial $5 offering can go, to how much can be given and received from sharing a testimony with others, to going to You in prayer instead of worrying about situations and watching you work it all out. I am truly forever in Your debt, and I have to do all that You ask of me to get right with You and be the person that You want me to be.

One of the best things that You have taught me is how to be in a relationship but still be able to put You first. I had a hard time doing that in the past. I can honestly say now that you are my first and only true love, second to no one and nothing. I love You so much and if it is in Your will, I can only ask that You never leave me. I have done so much in my past that You could have turned Your back on me long ago, but You are still here. Despite everything, You are still here, and I can't thank You enough.

Balancing work and fasting was no small feat. Energy levels dipped, and the aroma of "gourmet" lunches from colleagues became almost unbearable, even if it was just a simple sandwich. Yet, encouraging words from those around me and asking God for strength provided me with the endurance I needed.

One evening during my quiet time, I was jolted by a voice that I felt deep within my spirit—nonverbal but undeniably clear. It thundered, "Speak!" Just one word. My heart raced with questions: "Speak about what? To whom? When?" Silence enveloped me, leaving me with nothing but that single command from God. I kept this profound moment to myself, afraid that sharing it would lead to pressure to preach a sermon.

I felt closer to God than ever before, and for years, I yearned for that divine intimacy again.

As part of our preparation for the mission trip, the three of us sought the prayers of a woman bishop whom Jerelyn knew. After our introductions, the bishop and a group of women prayed fervently for our journey, asking for safe travels, effective delivery of the supplies, and the salvation of many souls. When it was my turn for prayer, the bishop placed a hand on my forehead and another on my stomach. She spoke words of prophecy over me, concluding with, "You will be an Esther in your life and for your people." I recognized Esther's name from the Bible but knew little else about her. Upon returning home, I eagerly read the entire book of Esther, hoping to uncover insights related to the prophecy.

Esther, an orphan raised by her cousin Mordecai, was groomed to become the queen. Her charm and courage allowed her to reveal her Jewish heritage, ultimately saving her people from genocide (Book of Esther, Chapters 1-10 NIV). However, after reading about her, I felt a disconnect. Esther's story seemed so distant from my own, and I set the prophecy aside, unsure of its significance.

A few days later, we visited Jerelyn's house to help pack the supplies. Her bedroom was overflowing with toiletries, baby items, clothes, and shoes. How would we fit all of this into just six pieces of luggage?

As we packed, Jerelyn opened up about the spiritual warfare she had faced during her fast. She described nights spent battling demonic spirits. Fear washed over me; the

I truly feel that I had gotten the closest to God than I had ever been before, and for years after, I would long for that experience again.

thought of such struggles made me want to retreat to the perceived safety of the world. It wasn't until years later, under the guidance of my pastor that I learned the truth: the enemy has no real power—Jesus conquered him at the Cross (Book of Colossians, Chapter 2, Verse 15 NIV). This revelation freed me to serve God wholeheartedly without the fear of physical attacks from the enemy.

The time for our trip finally arrived: September 25, 2004 – October 2, 2004. Each of us packed two large check-in bags filled with supplies, along with a carry-on for our clothes and toiletries. Checking in with Air Jamaica, our bags were overweight, but after Jerelyn explained our mission, we found favor with the airline staff and were allowed to check every bag without paying additional charges.

Having flown before, I thought I knew what to expect, but Air Jamaica surpassed all my previous experiences. Although we were not flying first class, I felt like a VIP. We were treated to complimentary drinks and a full meal—baked fish fillet, white rice, and mixed vegetables! It was a delightful start to my first trip to Jamaica.

Stepping off the plane, I experienced a profound culture shock. The contrast from Miami's skyscrapers and highways to Kingston's lush hills and unpaved roads left me awestruck. The taxi driver informed us that we had arrived at just the right time; the primary road from the airport had only recently reopened after being closed due to Hurricane Ivan's devastation.

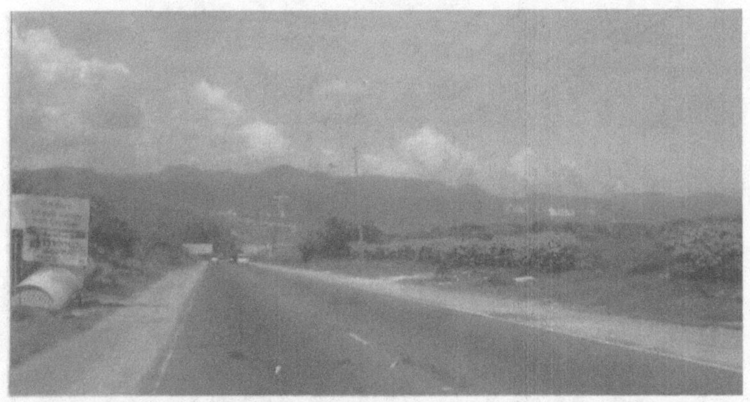

Roadway that was covered in beach sand and debris from Hurricane Ivan just a few days prior. Arriving in Kingston, Jamaica 2004

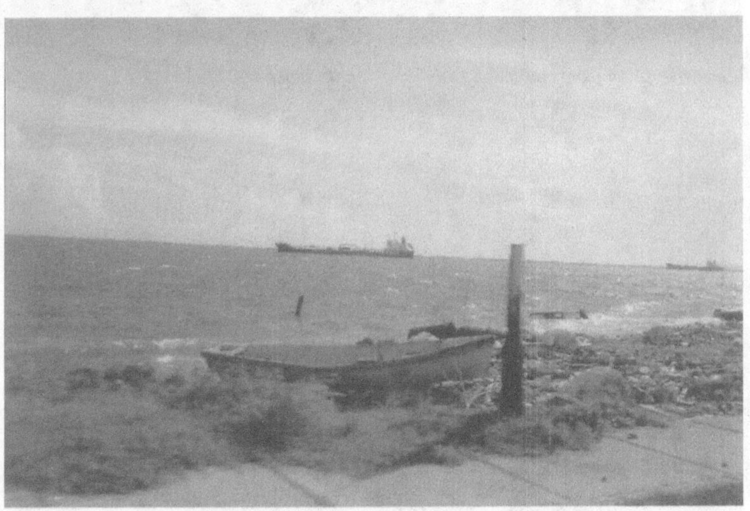

A boat on the beach. Kingston, Jamaica 2004

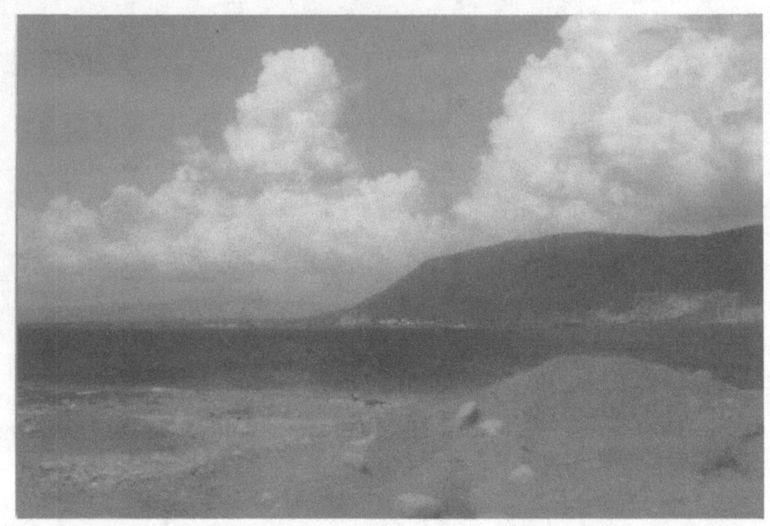

Beach disruption from Hurricane Ivan. Kingston, Jamaica 2004

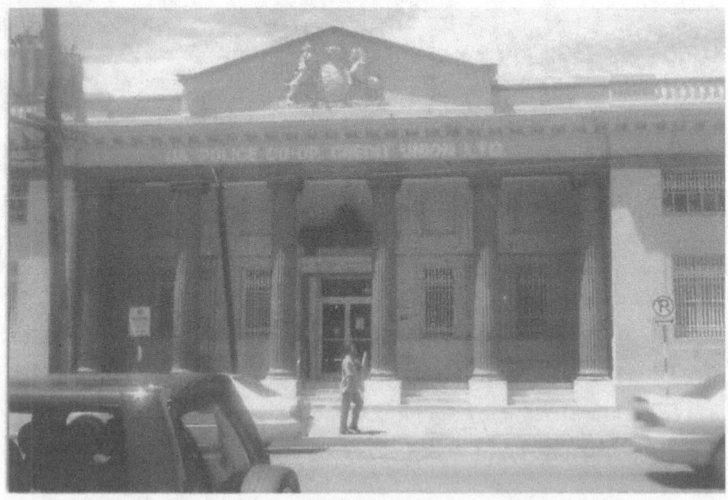

A police station and credit union in Kingston, Jamaica 2004

We stayed at the Hilton Hotel in Kingston 17, a slice of American comfort amidst the vibrant Jamaican backdrop.

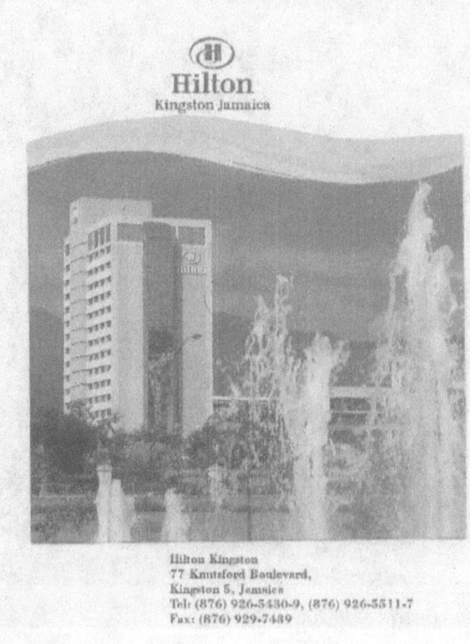

Hilton Kingston Hotel 2004

I had anticipated a brief trip focused solely on delivering supplies, but Jerelyn's heart was set on more. She was determined to share the gospel of Jesus Christ and lead others to salvation. We connected with the local church tasked with distributing the supplies to those in need.

Traveling about an hour and a half from the hotel on an unpaved road, we arrived at Unity Christian Centre on Commission Road in Kingston 2. The church was vibrant, with open doors and windows allowing the refreshing breeze to flow through. The congregation was warm and welcoming, and the children radiated joy, eagerly posing for photos.

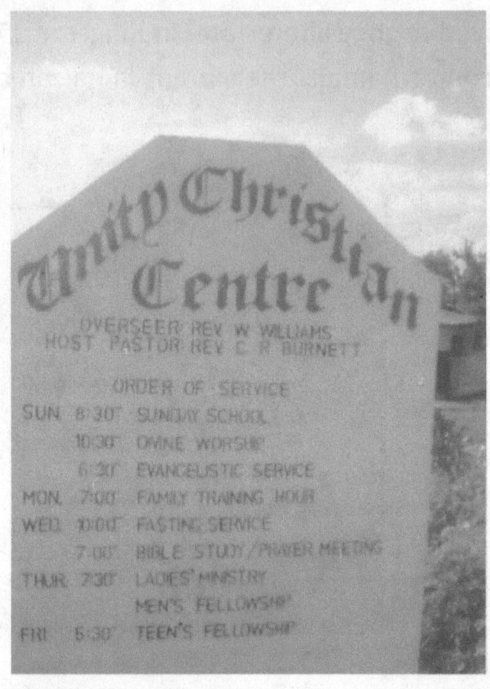

Unity Christian
Centre
OVERSEER: REV W WILLIAMS
HOST PASTOR: REV C R BURNETT
ORDER OF SERVICE
SUN 8:30 SUNDAY SCHOOL
10:30 DIVINE WORSHIP
6:30 EVANGELISTIC SERVICE
MON. 7:00 FAMILY TRAINING HOUR
WED. 10:00 FASTING SERVICE
7:00 BIBLE STUDY/PRAYER MEETING
THUR. 7:30 LADIES' MINISTRY
MEN'S FELLOWSHIP
FRI 5:30 TEEN'S FELLOWSHIP

Unity Christian Centre Sign 2004

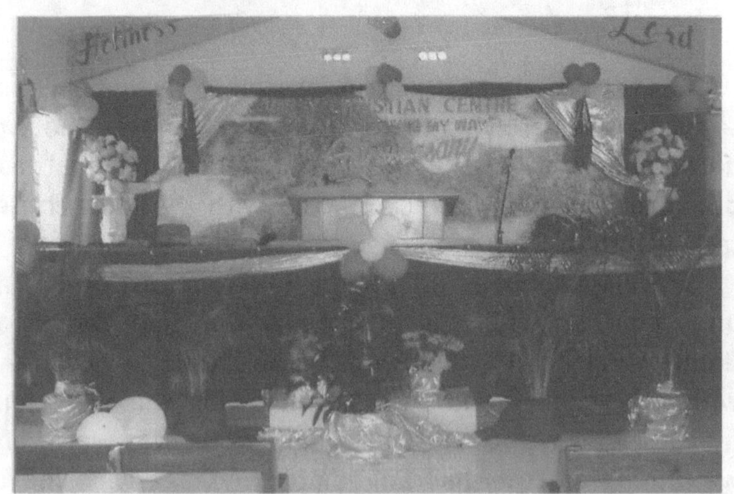

Unity Christian Centre Alter

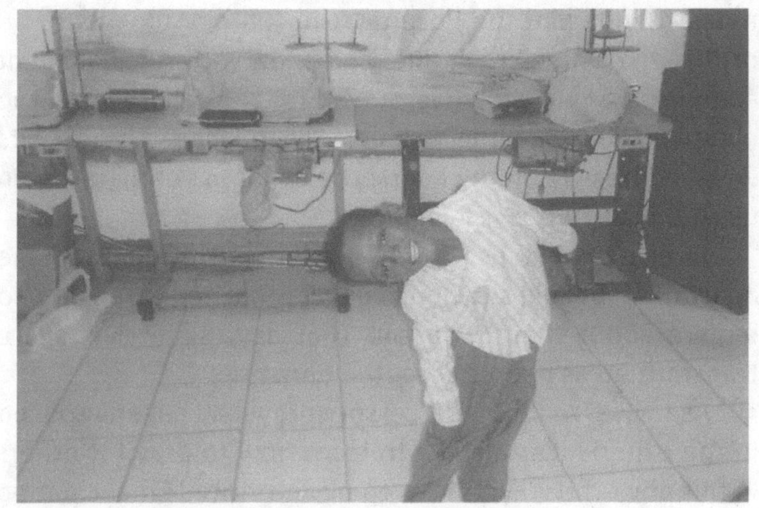

Happy kid at Unity Christian Centre

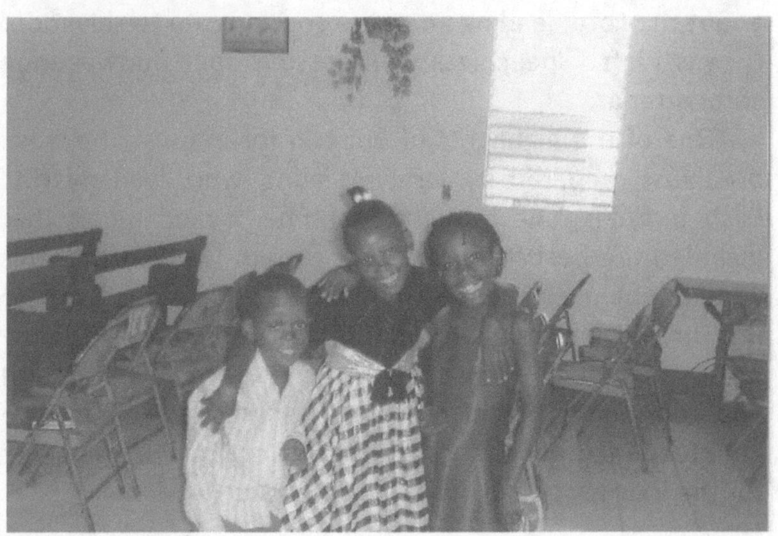

Happy kids at Unity Christian Centre

The next day, we accompanied Jerelyn to pick up a nurse friend from the hospital. Our journey took us to an orphanage, an elderly home, and a low-income apartment complex. At each stop, we prayed for the children and the elderly, asking for their safety and healing. These visits weighed heavily on my heart; the children yearned to join us, and many were visibly unwell.

Jerelyn's boldness in her faith was evident at the apartment building, where she approached strangers to inquire about their salvation. That day, many lives were transformed as people accepted Christ.

As I observed the intercessory prayers, I eagerly soaked in the experience, wishing to learn how to pray for others in this powerful way. One evening, we visited Emancipation Park to relax and appreciate Jamaica's beauty, yet Jerelyn was relentless. She engaged every passerby in conversation about the Lord, leading an entire soccer team to salvation. I was left speechless, witnessing her unwavering commitment.

One of the highlights of our trip for me was the fresh breakfast prepared by Jerelyn's aunt, who lived nearby. Each morning, she brought us home-cooked meals that included the best fish I had ever tasted. I vowed that this wouldn't be my last encounter with such delicious food.

Through this mission trip, I discovered not only the joy of serving others but also the transformative power of faith and community. Each moment strengthened my resolve and deepened my relationship with God, setting the stage for the journey ahead.

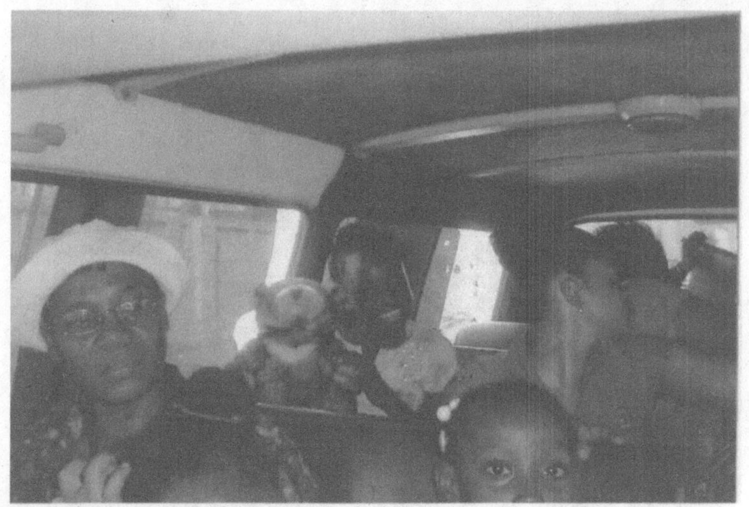

Jerelyn's nurse friend along for the day.

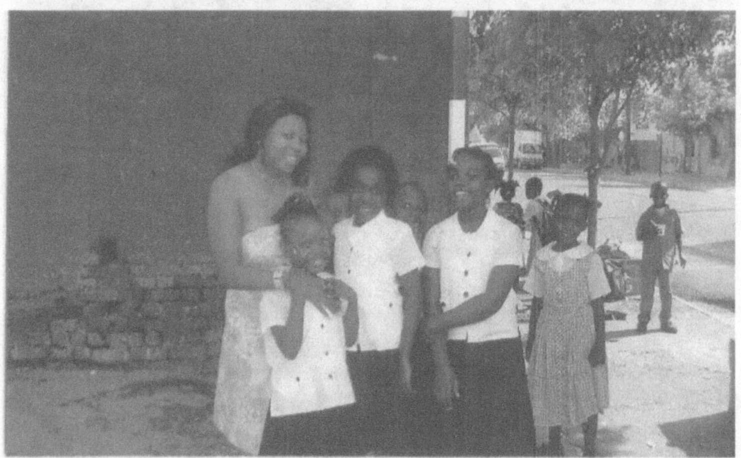

Jerelyn with orphan kids we prayed with

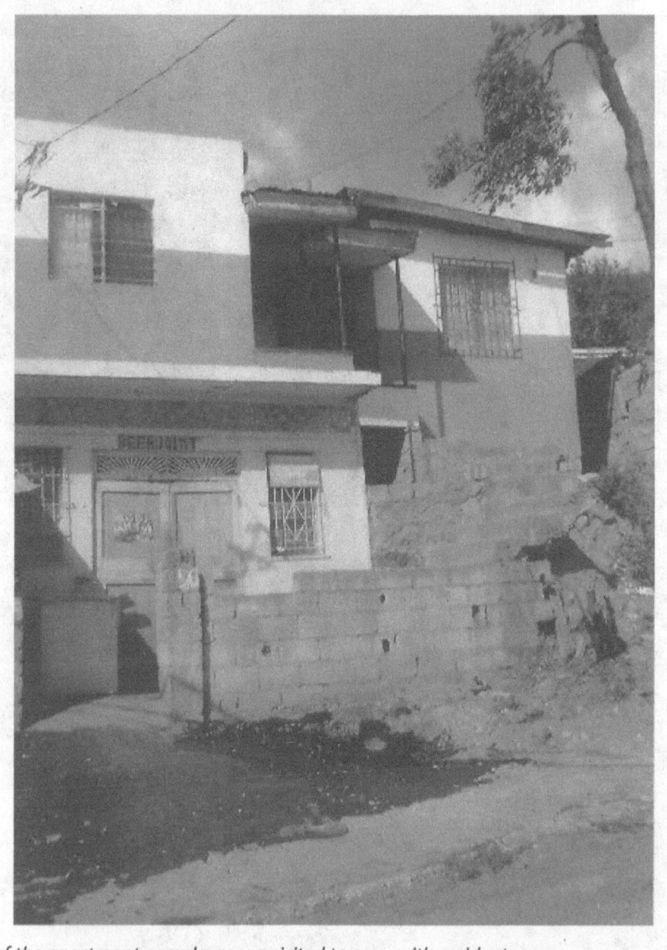

One of the apartment complexes we visited to pray with residents

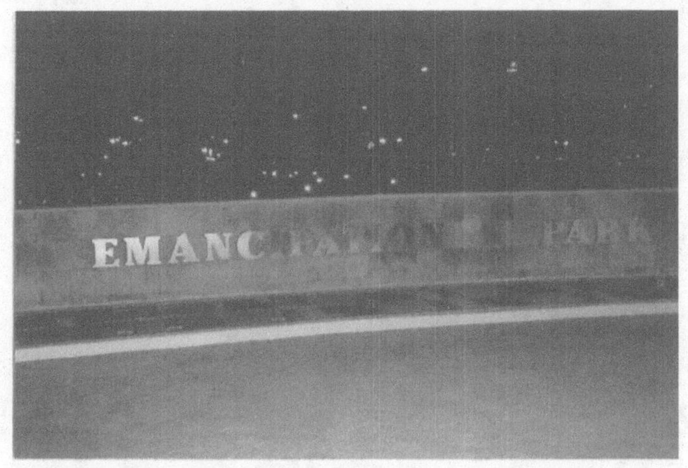

Emancipation Park Sign 2004

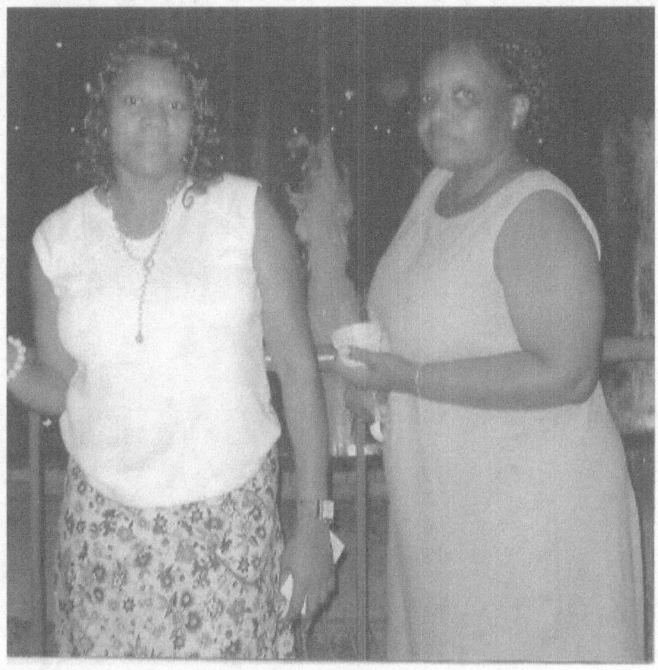

Jerelyn and Dr. Corridon at Emancipation Park 2004

Then I heard the voice of the Lord saying,
'Whom shall I send? And who will go for us?'
And I said, 'Here am I. Send me!'

-Isaiah 6:8

Let's Chat About It:
A Journey to Jamaica

1. What resonated with you the most about my journey to Jamaica? Were there specific moments that stood out to you?
2. How did I interpret the command to "speak"? Do you think it's important for individuals to recognize and act on such calls in their own lives?
3. I participated in a 10-day Daniel Fast. Have you ever fasted or engaged in a spiritual discipline? What was your experience like?
4. How do you think travel can impact one's worldview, especially in a faith context?
5. Discuss the significance of community support as shown in the chapter, particularly through prayers and fellowship with others. How does community enhance individual spiritual journeys?
6. I express fear regarding spiritual warfare. How do you relate to the concept of fear in spiritual contexts? How can one find courage in faith?
7. What did the prophecy regarding Esther mean to me, and how does it connect to the broader theme of identity and purpose in the chapter?

If this chapter connected with you, I'd love to hear about it! Share your thoughts by leaving a book review on Amazon.com.

3.
Faith Under Fire

When I returned home from my trip on October 3, 2004, I was on a spiritual high. The journey had blessed me beyond measure, and I was determined to carry forward the practices that had drawn me so close to God. I vowed to shield myself from negativity, focusing my heart and attitude solely on Him. Little did I know this commitment would soon face its first test.

That test arrived swiftly at work. Upon my return, I was met with a wave of negativity from the school's administration. Just two months earlier, I had celebrated a promotion from Microsystems Technician to Computer Specialist, a recognition of my hard work and dedication. Yet now, it felt as though nothing I did was right in my boss's eyes. Each day brought new, arbitrary tasks that contradicted the projects I had been assigned the day before, leaving me confused and frustrated.

In my role as a Microsystems Technician, I was responsible for installing, managing, and troubleshooting computers and networks across the school's campus. As a Computer Specialist, I not only retained these duties but also facilitated training sessions and provided technical support to instructors, staff, and students. My interactions with students of varying physical and mental abilities were especially fulfilling, as I took pride in ensuring that all assistive technologies functioned seamlessly.

However, the constant shifting of priorities took a toll on my health. I developed a mild case of carpal tunnel syndrome and had to wear a wrist brace to prevent further injury. Strangely, it seemed that once I donned the brace, my principal administrator began assigning me the physically demanding task of moving desktop computers from one classroom to another—only to have me reverse the process the next day. This behavior felt not only inconsiderate but also dismissive of my well-being. Eventually, I reached my breaking point. I thought, "There's no way God intended for me to be treated this way." Fueled by that conviction, I submitted my letter of resignation.

My principal administrator attempted to convince me to take a leave of absence instead, but I stood firm. I believed God was leading me away from this toxic environment, and so I walked away. My colleagues expressed sadness at my departure, but they respected my decision and, in time, many of them left the school as well.

Two weeks later, I found myself unemployed, with ample time to deepen my relationship with God and await His guidance for my next steps. I was completely reliant on Him when I faced my second test—a test of faith.

On October 31, 2004, I awoke to a beautiful day, eager to run errands. As I opened my apartment door, I was immediately halted by a shocking sight: a small wooden bowl filled with baby chicks with broken necks laying at my feet. My instincts screamed that this was no Halloween prank. I immediately cried out, "The blood of Jesus!" and slammed my door shut.

As I paced my living room floor, I kept pleading the blood of Jesus. Anger, fear and confusion gripped me. What did this mean? Why would someone do such a thing? I hadn't harmed anyone—why was this happening to me?

Gradually, I began to calm down and resolved to call the apartment building's emergency maintenance service to have the bowl removed. The maintenance worker assured me he would handle it immediately. I refused to leave my apartment until the bowl was gone; I would not allow evil of any kind to enter my space.

Shortly after my call for assistance, the maintenance person knocked. He informed me that an elderly woman who lived at the end of the hall, experienced in dealing with such matters, had come to inspect the bowl. She had spoken over it and disposed of it "properly," assuring him that whatever had occurred was not meant for me but for the tenant who lived there before I did. Though I thanked him, my worry lingered.

Determined to protect my home, I grabbed a bottle of oil from my kitchen and ventured into the hallway. With my apartment door closed, I splashed oil on the door and the ground where the bowl had been, all the while pleading the blood of Jesus aloud. I then mopped the oil around the ground near my door, not caring if anyone passing by thought I was crazy. I didn't know if my actions would have any effect, but they felt necessary. Exhausted and sweaty, I discarded the mop and retreated inside, praying for God's protection. I believed He heard my plea, and my worries gradually subsided. That night, I slept soundly.

Two months later, I completed my coursework at Barry University, earning a Master of Science degree in Information Technology. In January 2005, I started a new job at DirecTV. As I was finishing up my three-month probationary period and awaited the activation of my medical benefits in March, life was looking up. I was

I was completely dependent on Him, trusting that every test was preparing me for something greater.

working but I also had time to spend with God. I had been growing my hair out naturally for the past two years, embracing who I was, and honoring the way God made me. Yet, unbeknownst to me, my most challenging test was looming.

In an unexpected turn, my apartment became infested with mold. The bathroom's broken ventilation fan, combined with a leaking pipe in the wall, led to a mold outbreak in my walk-in closet, which shared a wall with the bathroom. This was my first apartment, and I hadn't understood the importance of proper ventilation, especially in a room with no window. My closet was filled with memories—photo albums, scrapbooks, clothes, and shoes—all ruined by mold.

I reported the issue to the rental office, and they promised to "clean" my apartment with a mold-killing substance. I knew there was no real solution without fixing the ventilation fan and the leaking pipe. A short time later, the mold returned. When I returned to the rental office to request a transfer to another apartment, I overheard another tenant, a mother of three, pleading for help due to mold affecting her child's asthma. The employee dismissed her concerns, but my request for a move was granted, probably because a one-bedroom apartment was available. Outraged for that mother, I resolved to act. I called the Environmental Protection Agency (EPA) for assistance, only to learn that they had no authority over apartment buildings, leaving it up to property owners to address mold infestations as they saw fit. I was left astonished by this news.

Consider it pure joy, my brothers and sisters, whenever you face trials of many kinds, because you know that the testing of your faith produces perseverance. Let perseverance finish its work so that you may be mature and complete, not lacking anything.

-James 1:2-4

Let's Chat About It:
Faith Under Fire

1. How does my experience with the toxic work environment reflect my commitment to faith and resilience? What would you have done in my situation?

2. I face both physical and spiritual challenges throughout the chapter. How do you think these different types of tests contribute to my personal growth?

3. What role does faith play in my decision to leave my job and navigate the unsettling spiritual encounter at my apartment? How would you have handled the situation with the bowl outside the door?

4. I make a strong connection between my relationship with God and my decision to embrace my natural hair. What do you think this decision symbolizes in the broader context of my faith journey?

5. How does my response to the mold infestation and the lack of support from my rental office reveal my evolving sense of personal power and resilience?

6. Which moment in the chapter stood out to you as the most challenging for me, and why? How do you think my faith helped me persevere?

Was there a moment in this chapter that spoke to you? I would be honored if you left a book review on Amazon.com and shared your experience.

4.
Through the Valley of the Shadows

The Miami sun blazed down as I shifted heavy furniture from one apartment to the other. Fatigue set in early, but I shrugged it off as exhaustion from the heat and humidity. I focused on staying hydrated, but despite the bottles of water and juice I consumed, my thirst remained unquenchable. Even worse, I wasn't using the restroom as often as usual. By evening, my body refused to cooperate; I was regurgitating any food I tried to eat.

A friend stopped by with food and an offer to help. Gratefully, I accepted, but nothing I ate stayed down. Still, I convinced myself it was just the strain of moving combined with the relentless Miami heat. As the weekend wore on, I decided to wait until Monday to visit a medical clinic. Without health insurance, an emergency room visit was out of the question.

Monday came, and after hours of waiting, the clinic ran blood tests and handed me some antibiotics, suggesting I return in two weeks if my symptoms persisted. The weeks passed, and not only did the antibiotics fail to help, but my condition worsened. My ankles were swollen to the size of elephant legs, and I felt utterly depleted. Deep down, I knew something was gravely wrong.

In desperation, I drove to my parents' house and asked my mom to take me to the emergency room. It was quite far away, and I didn't feel safe driving that far in my condition. I arrived at the emergency room at around noon on a day in February. I checked in, my vital signs were taken, and I was ushered into the chaotic ER waiting room. Because I did not have medical insurance I was not seen right away. I sat in the waiting room for hours. I didn't eat, drink, sleep, or use the restroom because I was afraid I wouldn't hear my name called and miss my turn. Also, I would have lost my seat in a crowded emergency room and would have had to stand on these elephant ankles until I was seen. I was in agony. I was cold and I couldn't get comfortable in the plastic chair I was sitting in but also grateful that I had an uncomfortable seat to sit in compared to those who had been standing for hours. The room buzzed with the sounds of hacking coughs, cries of pain, and frustrated outbursts. I really wanted to sleep, but I had to stay awake in case my name was called to be seen by a doctor. No one waited with me; no one besides my parents even knew I was there. After a few hours, my parents stopped calling to get updates. They probably assumed I was being treated. I had never felt so alone and invaluable in my life. And in that long, torturous wait, the thought crossed my mind that maybe it wouldn't be so bad to simply close my eyes and never wake up. Finally, at 10:30 the next morning, a doctor called my name. She was furious when she discovered no one had informed me that my bloodwork, taken weeks earlier, showed dangerously high creatinine levels. My kidneys were failing, and the medical staff was amazed I had survived those two weeks. The urgency in the room shifted; suddenly, after 22 hours of waiting, it was an emergency. I was laughing on the inside at the irony. I was rushed to a gurney, and finally, I could sleep without fear of missing my turn. So, I slept.

When I woke, I was surrounded by machines, tubes, and nurses monitoring every aspect of my health. The diagnosis was end-stage renal failure. My creatinine levels were nine times higher than normal. As the medical team scrambled to stabilize me, I realized how close I had come to the brink.

According to the Mayo Clinic (2023) a creatinine test is a measure of how well kidneys are performing their job of filtering waste from blood. Creatinine is a chemical compound left over from energy-producing processes in muscles. Healthy kidneys filter creatinine out of the blood. Creatinine exits the body as a waste product in urine. A measurement of creatinine in blood or urine provides clues to help doctors determine how well the kidneys are working (Mayo Clinic, 2023). Serum creatinine is reported as milligrams of creatinine to a deciliter of blood (mg/dL) or micromoles of creatinine to a liter of blood (micromoles/L). The typical range for serum creatinine for adult men is 0.74 to 1.35 mg/dL and for adult women, 0.59 to 1.04 mg/dL (Mayo Clinic, 2023). My creatinine level was over 9.0. Both of my kidneys were functioning at 10% out of 100.

It would take another two weeks and a half in the hospital for the doctors to get me stable and agree on a medical treatment plan. There is so much that can happen in a hospital in two and a half weeks' time.

I was in a hospital room that held two beds divided by a curtain. My bed was on the window side of the room, the other bed was on the door side of the room. You'd think that there would be a nice view, but looking between the thick window bars and screens, all I could see was the towering building next door. Bummer.

I never got to meet my roommate. The curtain was always drawn, and she always moaned in pain. One night, at about 3 am, lights, panic, and noise filled our room. She was dying. Medical staff rushed her away. The next day, I got another roommate. A man this time. His family came to visit him throughout the days. I never heard his voice. It was as if his family was holding a vigil. There was always someone there with him at all times. Then one night, I was awakened by loud outcries and yelling. It was his family. My roommate had died.

The next morning, a charge nurse came by to see me. She asked how my stay had been so far and if I was comfortable. I immediately expressed that I was in fact uncomfortable with patients dying around me every night. I started to think that death might mistakenly visit my bed next. She apologized for my experience and said she would see what she could do. I didn't expect to see her again or for anything to change. A few hours later, however, a nurse kindly moved me into a private room, where I found peace. I spent hours watching the Trinity Broadcasting Network, drawing strength from the spiritual nourishment it provided. Friends, family, and sorority sisters visited me, filling my room with love and support. The consistency of the calls, visits, and get-well cards from my sorority sisters during this time really helped my parents gain a better understanding of and appreciation for the sisterhood, as they were completely against me joining during my undergraduate school years. As the days wore on, the visits became less frequent. I was left alone with my thoughts—and with God.

It was during one of these reflective moments that I realized that through everything I had been experiencing, I had not been afraid. The spirit of fear never came over me. I was amazed at this revelation because I had almost died. If I had remained at home for a few more days without coming to get treatment, my body would have poisoned itself by retaining all of the toxins that kidneys help to expel from the body, and I would have been dead. It was at that moment that God allowed me to reflect back to the 10-day fast that I completed just a few months before. That time with Him had prepared me not only for the mission trip to Jamaica, but also for such a time as this. I thanked Him for the revelation, and I was at peace with my current situation, although I didn't understand it fully at the time.

There is not always much awareness of time and space while being a patient in the hospital for an extended period. There are no calendars, and back then there was no jewelry allowed, including watches. Days began to run into each other and the only way to really gauge time is by when meals were delivered and when shifts changed for the nurses. The chemical cocktails that were being served through my veins via IV and also with meals in pill form didn't help either. I mention this to say that I don't know when it began...

It was a Saturday. I was trying to wake up, but I couldn't open my eyes. It was as if my eyelids were glued shut, but I could see the light from my bed shine through the skin of my eyelids. Panic set in when I realized I couldn't move. I tried to yell, but no sound came out. Then, I heard a voice—a low, male voice telling me to sleep, assuring me that everything would be okay. "I don't want to sleep!" I heard myself say. “I want to wake up!” “Just relax. Everything will be okay. Just sleep,” the voice said. I fought against it, crying out in my mind that I didn’t want to sleep, that I wanted to live. And then, just like that, the voice and the light were gone. I knew in my heart that there was no actual person that had spoken to me. And as loudly as I yelled, I knew that I had never actually said a word.

I woke up sometime later, disoriented, and looking around the room. It was the same calm and peaceful room, but something was different. My mom sat at my bedside, looking exhausted, sad, and concerned. I asked her if she was okay and of course she said yes. She would have said yes either way, so I didn’t quite believe her answer. I knew that I had been asleep for some time so I thought it might be the next day by now. “Mom, it’s Sunday, right?” I asked her, just to be sure. “No sweetheart, it’s Wednesday,” she answered. “Wednesday! Well, where did Sunday, Monday, and Tuesday go?” I exclaimed. “You don’t remember?” she said, “You had an adverse reaction to the medication you were given, and the nurse had to come in and restrain you in order for the doctors to perform a procedure. You were irate and yelling for your dad. ‘I want my daddy. I want my daddy’ is what you kept yelling. They eventually had to strap your arms and legs to the bed.” I was shocked. “Are you serious? I don’t remember any of that!” I said in response. For months afterwards I tried to search my memory for even a glimpse of the events that my mom had described. To this day, I have yet to remember.

If you know someone who is in the hospital right now, please visit them, call them, or send them a card.

I truly believe that what I thought was a dream actually happened. I believe that I was fighting for my life in some spiritual realm. I believe that the male voice I heard was that of the enemy trying to persuade me into an eternal sleep, but I was not ready to leave this earth.

A few days later I was still contemplating what I had experienced. No one knew what happened but me. People might think that I was crazy if I told them. People might say that the medicine caused a hallucination. But I know the truth. God spared my life that day. But why? I must have a purpose that hasn't been met yet. I haven't been obedient to God's Word. So why me? I didn't deserve to be spared. Then I remembered what I heard when I was fasting. *Speak*. That's it. God gave me a Word and maybe He spared my life because I'm supposed to speak about something. But what? I was so confused.

As I've said, there is a lot of time to spend with your thoughts while in the hospital. At one point, I began to reflect on the life that I had lived thus far. After all, I almost died. What would have happened if I had died? What would people remember about me? My two degrees? My many hours spent working at my jobs? The community service I've done? I don't have a husband or children... who would miss me? What mark on the world have I left? I would've died without experiencing true love. The kind of real love between a man and a woman. This revelation made me cry.

It was at that point I realized everything I had been busying myself with didn't really matter much. If I left the earth right now, there wouldn't be much to show for my life. That was a depressing thought. I vowed to make *people* priority over working a job and going to school. Building relationships and helping others would be most important to me. I would spend more time traveling and enjoying the beautiful places God has created on the earth. I asked God to please not let me leave this earth without experiencing true love. I believed God would honor my request.

If you know someone who is in the hospital right now, please visit them, call them, or send them a card. The hospital is much like what I imagine prison to be in that after a while you begin to feel like people have forgotten about you and their lives have gone on without you. This is when thoughts of unworthiness, sadness, loneliness, and "no one will miss me if I'm gone" start to creep in. This is when some people start to feel tired of fighting and want to give up on the fight for their lives. It is at these times that I believe a spirit gives up. But if family, friends, and loved ones keep visiting, calling, sending cards, sending flowers, sending gifts, and sending snacks, it helps people remember that they are loved and cherished. It will help their spirit be happy and motivated to continue to fight; "There is a reason to keep fighting because there are people out there who love me."

I decided that it would be selfish of me to give up on my life. All the people who had invested their time and energy into me would be let down... my parents, my family, my friends, my teachers... they've all worked so hard with me, poured so much of themselves into me. For me to willingly leave now would be a waste of their investment in me. If I gave up, it may send them the message that what they did for me didn't matter and that might influence them to pour less into someone else. I am not okay with that. So, I will continue on.

Perhaps the most painful thing that I experienced during my two- week stay in the hospital happened shortly before my discharge. Shifts had changed for the evening nurses to start work. One night, I got a younger Hispanic man as my overnight nurse. He came in to administer my final bag of intravenous liquid medication for the evening. It is usually set to slow drip for a few hours until the bag is empty. Shortly after he'd left the room, I began to feel pain in my arm. Initially I thought it was because I had had the IV in for so long, maybe my arm was just irritated. The pain increased. As time went by, the pain became so bad that I felt like my veins were on fire. I hit the button for my nurse to come back and check it out for me. He came, I explained, he checked the equipment and said that everything was fine and there was nothing more he could do. I asked if there was anyone else available to double check it. He said no. I believed him because the night shift is usually more lightly staffed than the day shift. He left my room. The pain got so intense that I felt like my vein was going to explode at any moment. The pain was so bad that I began to cry. I couldn't do anything else but cry. I cried for over four hours until the medicine was done.

My friend had come by to see how I was doing. I explained what was happening. He just sat next to me and rubbed my back as I cried. I didn't want him to see me crying, but pain trumped pride in that moment.

The next morning after the medical shifts changed, a new nurse came in. She asked how my night was, and I shared my ordeal with her. She checked the machine where all the previous settings were still stored. She observed that the previous nurse set the liquid flow speed too high. So instead of it being set to a slow drip, the medicine had been racing through my veins. She apologized profusely for his error, and I just could not stop thinking about how the most excruciating pain I had ever felt could have been prevented. I spent two and a half weeks in the hospital before I was released to go home. I am thankful for the family, friends, and church members who interceded in prayer on my behalf during that time.

I thank God for my fasting and TBN experiences before my health failed. I believe that time of growing closer to God helped me to not fear for my life during this time. There was a peace that I had throughout the entire ordeal that I know I probably would not have had without my newly developed relationship with Him. I am so grateful.

During the time I spent in the hospital, there was a lot going on outside. Bills were coming due, and I hadn't been able to go to work. My parents took documents to the apartment rental office to inform them of my whereabouts. My parents asked the manager to waive the rent that was currently due and to release me without penalty from my rental agreement. I had only lived there for nine months, and my lease was for a year. The manager initially resisted the requests, but my parents reminded them of the mold issue I had been having in their building and also mentioned that the doctors were unsure as to what caused my current sickness. With those words, the manager agreed to all terms.

A couple of days after I had been admitted into the hospital, my parents took hospital documentation to my manager at work and explained my situation. She thanked them for informing her and said that my job would be waiting for me when I got better. About two weeks after my discharge from the hospital, I went to speak with my manager regarding when I should return to work. When I got to my workplace, I was promptly referred to her boss, and I was told that I had been fired due to poor attendance. I asked if they were aware of the hospital documentation that was shared previously. They said yes and maintained that I was fired anyway.

I was crushed, devastated, and angry at the injustice. How could I be fired for something that was completely out of my control, especially when I did what I could to provide documentation for my absence? But I couldn't dwell on that. Now I had to focus on my recovery and figure out how to move forward.

For the next few months, I visited doctors frequently to monitor my recovery and to discuss my next steps. I went to nephrologists (renal/kidney doctors) and arthritis doctors on a regular basis. My nephrologist informed me that at some point in the future, I would have to start dialysis. He was a young doctor, maybe even a resident, and the way he described dialysis was mortifying to me. I was not happy about this at all. The doctor also informed me that there were two medicines that I could take in the meantime to stabilize my renal function, Cellcept and Prednisone. Each medication would essentially work for one year each before the side effects would outweigh the benefits of taking them. So, I had at least two years before having to start dialysis.

I spent the summer visiting doctors, recovering at my parents' house, and worrying about what I would do with myself. I felt fine. The meds were working well. I was 25 years old.

During this time, I received a bill in the mail from the hospital for around nineteen thousand dollars for the time that I was there.

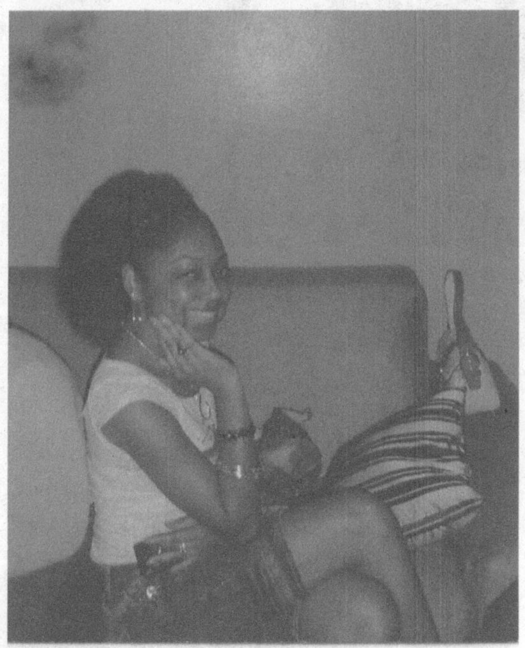

One of the side effects of Prednisone is puffy or blowfish like cheeks.

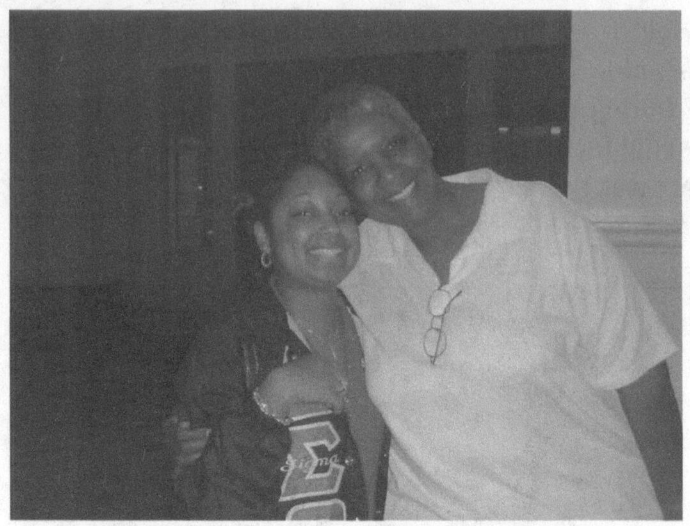

One of the side effects of Prednisone is puffy or blowfish like cheeks.

So do not fear, for I am with you; do not be dismayed, for I am your God. I will strengthen you and help you; I will uphold you with my righteous right hand.

-Isaiah 41:10

Let's Chat About It: Through the Valley of the Shadows

1. I describe a moment of intense loneliness in the hospital waiting room. Have you ever experienced a moment where you felt invisible or forgotten in a critical situation? How did you cope?
2. How does my journey highlight the intersection of physical vulnerability, spiritual awareness, and the search for purpose?
3. Reflect on the significance of the hospital room experiences with other patients. How do these encounters with death shape my perspective on my own life and future?
4. I mention a spiritual experience, a voice encouraging me to sleep forever. How do you interpret this moment? Do you believe it was a supernatural event, or could it have been something else?
5. Health disparities are subtly referenced when I describe my long wait due to lack of medical insurance. How does this experience reflect broader issues in the healthcare system? What might the author be suggesting about the importance of advocacy?
6. What do you want your legacy to be? And how does that align with how you live today?

If this chapter connected with you, I'd love to hear about it! Share your thoughts by leaving a book review on Amazon.com.

5.
Resilience in Transition

In July 2005, the phone rang with an opportunity I hadn't anticipated. Soror Gwendolyn Bryant, newly appointed as principal of Earlington Heights Elementary School, called me with exciting news. She was assembling her new team for the upcoming school year and wanted me to be part of it. With a warm familiarity in her voice, she asked about my well-being before offering me a position that took me by surprise: Instructional Technology Specialist. My heart leaped. This wasn't just a job offer; it was the very role my mentor, Gardenia Bulluck, held at Biscayne Gardens Elementary. Having worked closely with Gardenia, I knew the role inside out. It felt like another prayer answered, exceeding what I'd imagined.

The school year kicked off in August, and for the next two years, I thrived. I enjoyed my work, my health was stable, and I found fulfillment in my new responsibilities. Yet, despite this, there was a shadow lingering in the background—my doctors' periodic mentions of dialysis. Each time they brought it up, I declined. The concept of dialysis was too overwhelming, too foreign. I didn't want to confront it or fully understand its implications. Fear and uncertainty made me avoid the topic altogether, as if ignoring it might somehow keep it at bay.

During a quiet lunch one day, a friend and colleague asked me a question that completely shifted the conversation: "Are you angry that this has happened to you?" I paused, thinking about the question. "No," I replied, "I wouldn't wish this experience on anyone, but if my going through it spares someone else from having to endure it, then I'm okay with it." Her reaction, a simple "Wow," showed me the power of resilience I'd been cultivating, even when I hadn't recognized it.

By June 2007, Gwen reached her own milestone: retirement. I was genuinely happy for her—proud of her accomplishment. But as much as I celebrated her success, I sensed a shift on the horizon. At her retirement party, the atmosphere was bittersweet. We all wished her well, but there was an unspoken understanding that things would never be the same. Over the next three years, we welcomed two new principals.

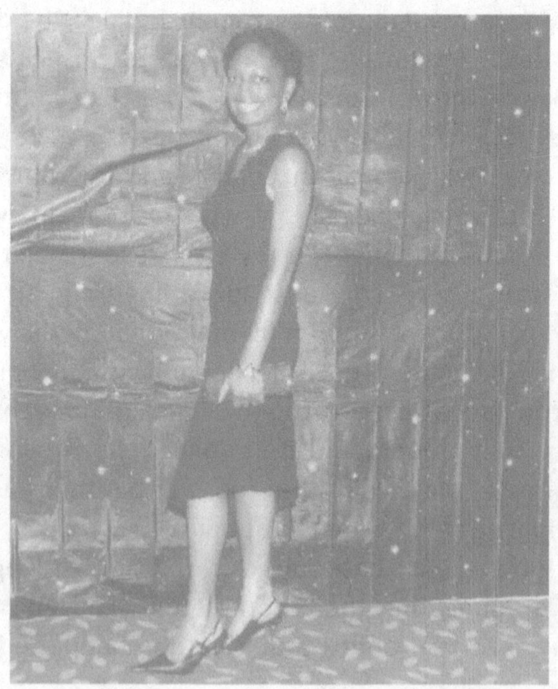

Neither possessed the steady leadership and warmth Gwen had embodied, and under their tenure, my experiences at the school steadily declined. The joy I'd found in my role was fading.

Meanwhile, my health was also shifting. The two-year period my medications were supposed to hold strong was ending. I met with my young renal doctor, hoping for a clear next step. Instead, he offered a vague plan: "We'll just monitor you and make adjustments as needed." It was a hollow reassurance. The reality was glaringly obvious—I was getting sicker, and without the proper treatment, it was only a matter of time before something terrible could happen.

I couldn't believe this was the plan: wait and watch my health deteriorate. But what could I do? I returned home, resigned to the inevitable, as my body started to show signs of decline.

This chapter of my life was marked by transitions: some filled with promise, others fraught with uncertainty. Yet, through it all, I learned that resilience isn't just about bouncing back from challenges; it's about enduring, even when the path ahead is unclear.

”

Resilience isn’t just about bouncing back from challenges; it’s about enduring, even when the path ahead is unclear.

The Lord himself goes before you and will be with you; he will never leave you nor forsake you. Do not be afraid; do not be discouraged."

-Deuteronomy 31:8

Let's Chat About It:
Resilience in Transition

1. How do you think my relationship with Soror Gwendolyn Bryant influenced my career path at this stage?
2. What role does mentorship play in shaping my confidence and success in my new position?
3. I express fear and denial about starting dialysis. How do you think fear of the unknown can affect major health decisions? Have you ever experienced a similar hesitation?
4. What emotions do I convey when reflecting on my declining health and the medical advice I received? How would you have reacted in my situation?
5. How does my faith contribute to my resilience throughout the challenges I face, both professionally and personally?
6. In the chapter, I mention that I would rather endure hardship than wish it on someone else. How does this selfless mindset shape my outlook on my health struggles?
7. How do I cope with the shifting dynamics at work and my health concerns at the same time? How do resilience and adaptability come into play in both areas?
8. How does my reflection on this period of my life help frame the larger themes of resilience and growth in my story?

Did this chapter move you in some way? I'd love to read your thoughts—please leave a review on Amazon.

6.
A New Experience

The hospital room felt cold and sterile, but it was the urgency in the doctors' eyes that made the walls close in. An emergency catheter had to be installed in my neck, a thin tube that would be my lifeline as I began dialysis. It marked the beginning of a whirlwind I wasn't ready for—one filled with new medical terms, endless paperwork, and procedures I'd never imagined.

Dialysis. The word itself carried weight, like a stone in my chest. My kidneys had failed me, no longer filtering my blood as they should. The Cleveland Clinic (2021) describes dialysis clinically: a treatment to remove waste and excess fluid from the bloodstream. But the reality was far less detached. Dialysis was personal, invasive, and deeply emotional. When given the choice, I opted for hemodialysis at a center instead of trying to navigate peritoneal dialysis at home. I wanted professionals around me—I needed the security of knowing I was in capable hands.

Before my first treatment, I faced another procedure: the creation of an arteriovenous fistula. It is a surgical connection between an artery and vein in my right arm, meant to ease access for dialysis. Although some people have an arteriovenous graft installed, which is a soft, hollow tube that connects the artery and vein, I had an arteriovenous fistula installed which means the surgeon connected an artery and vein together in my arm. AV fistulas and grafts enlarge the connected artery and vein, which makes dialysis access easier. They also help blood flow in and out of [the] body faster during dialysis treatments (Cleveland Clinic, 2021). The decision to use my right arm, rather than my dominant left, seemed trivial, but in situations like this, every detail mattered. I was left waiting for weeks as my arm healed, my body preparing for the battle ahead.

Fear ruled those early days. Would the catheter cause an infection? Would the fistula surgery go wrong? The possibility of blood clots, the pain of dialysis, even the thought of death loomed constantly. My mind was a persistent storm of "what ifs," leaving little room for peace. The unknown was overwhelming.

When I finally walked into DaVita Dialysis Center on February 28, 2008, the warmth of the receptionist felt like a lifeline in the sea of my apprehension. Her calm reassured not just me, but my parents, who were by my side, equally unsure of what this journey would entail. Nurse Greg Sage was assigned to me that day, and I later learned he was one of the best. His nurturing presence helped ease my fears as he connected me to the machine that would cleanse my blood, reassuring me that I was in good hands.

At first, the process was relatively painless. The catheter in my chest allowed for a simple connection to the machine, though its presence was a constant source of discomfort, especially when showering. When the fistula in my arm finally healed, I was relieved to have the catheter removed, just as an infection began to form. It was a narrow escape.

One of the biggest challenges at the start of each dialysis treatment was determining how much fluid to remove. My nurses and I had to play a delicate guessing game with my body weight, factoring in everything from my clothing to the last time I ate. Too much fluid removal would cause excruciating cramps, a pain that could bring anyone to their knees. But my nurses, with their skill and care, made sure we got it right most of the time. God's hand was evident in their precision and dedication.

High blood pressure became a constant battle, a side effect of my kidney failure (one of many). Each day felt like a tightrope walk, balancing medicines for potassium, phosphorus, iron, and blood pressure. It wasn't just the physical toll of managing these levels, but the mental load of remembering to take each pill at the right time, while still showing up for life, for work, and for myself. Some days I succeeded, other days I faltered. But through it all, I never stopped fighting. Every day, I wanted someone to understand what I was going through and send some love and support my way.

I can still remember the taste of the iron infusions during dialysis treatments—like bitter black licorice. The metallic tang was a small reminder of how far removed my life was from what it used to be. Along with the medical treatments came the harsh reality of a restricted diet. Low sodium. Low potassium. Low phosphorus. And worst of all, limited liquid intake. It was as if I had to relearn how to eat, turning the joy of a good meal into a math equation of nutrients I couldn't exceed.

Every day, I wanted someone to understand what I was going through and send some love and support my way.

Southern cooking, mostly made by my Dad, had been a staple of my life for 25 years, and suddenly, I was faced with bland food that made me long for a different reality. This was the time when reading nutrition facts on food labels was critical. The frustration of reading every nutrition label and the anger of missing out on meals I loved— weighed on me. Eating out was out of the question. My quality of life plummeted, not just because of the dialysis treatments, but because of the loss of simple pleasures like enjoying a meal.

Nurse Sage kept me accountable, his eyes catching the telltale signs in my bloodwork if I strayed from the prescribed diet. At times, the frustration boiled over, but eventually, I came to accept the changes. It took over a year, but by then, I'd made peace with my new normal. I learned to eat to live, not live to eat, and though the diet was no longer a necessity years later, it became a way of life for me. Even today, I check nutrition labels, staying mindful of what I put into my body.

That year of adjustment was more than just medical—it was spiritual, mental, and emotional. Each day was a step toward resilience, a fight to reclaim control in the face of something I couldn't escape. It wasn't easy, but it was my path. And through it all, God's presence was a constant, guiding me through the waters of dialysis and back into life.

Do not be anxious about anything, but in every situation, by prayer and petition, with thanksgiving, present your requests to God.

-Philippians 4:6

Let's Chat About It:
A New Experience

1. How does my experience with dialysis shape my perspective on life and resilience?

2. How does my relationship with Nurse Greg Sage reflect the importance of support systems in the midst of personal trials?

3. I reflect on learning to "eat to live, not live to eat." How does this shift in lifestyle represent deeper changes in my outlook on life?

4. How do faith and spirituality emerge as a source of strength in this chapter? Can you identify moments where your faith helps you cope?

5. What do you think I mean when I say I "wanted someone to understand what I was going through and send some love and support"? How does this sentiment resonate with you?

6. How might this chapter change the way readers think about chronic illness and the day-to-day challenges of managing health?

7. If you were in my position, what strategies or mindsets do you think would help you cope with such a life-altering situation?

If this chapter resonated with you, I'd be thrilled to hear your thoughts. Please consider sharing your review on Amazon.

7.
Resilient Heart

In my mid-to-late twenties, as I grappled with health challenges and maintained a full-time job, I was also wanting companionship. Like many women my age, I dreamed of marriage and building a family with a partner who would love me unconditionally—someone who could empathize with my struggles and support me through them. My prayers were for a solid partner with whom I could share my life, someone I could pour my love into.

However, what unfolded over those few years instead was a series of relationships that were interesting to say the least. One notable encounter was with a man I dated. On one of our dates, I noticed a tan line on his ring finger, and, upon inquiring, he revealed that he was in the midst of a divorce. He claimed that the divorce papers had been filed and they were merely waiting to be processed. While I found him attractive, I realized that his unresolved marriage was a dealbreaker for me. I expressed my willingness to date him after his divorce was finalized, and we parted ways. Some time later, he reached out to inform me that his divorce was complete, but he was no longer interested in dating me, feeling betrayed by my decision to end the relationship. We agreed to disagree.

My next relationship was with a handsome, charming man who exuded a bad-boy allure. Although we had little in common, I dismissed that as a barrier to exploring love. He was an aspiring rapper, spending countless hours in music studios, writing, and recording lyrics. I began to immerse myself in his world, even meeting his mother, a devoted deaconess at her church.

However, as time passed, I became aware of his troubling habits—street hustling, drinking, smoking marijuana, and a lack of stable employment. I noticed he lived with his mother and didn't own a car, but I refrained from judgment, believing everyone's journey is different. Yet, there were moments of mild verbal abuse that I ignored, brushing them aside as inconsequential.

Things took a drastic turn when he ended up in jail for an offense I can no longer recall. Each day, he pleaded with me by phone to bail him out, and when he called one evening to report a fight he was in where part of his ear had been bitten off, fear for his safety propelled me to action. Without knowing the process, I gathered what little money I had and managed to secure his release from the Miami jail, where I was greeted by the sight of his bandaged ear.

Fast forward to my own health crisis: I spent 22 hours in the emergency room and two weeks hospitalized, during which time he visited me. I felt a flicker of gratitude that he cared. But that gratitude quickly dissolved when, during the visit, he asked to borrow my car. I firmly refused, understanding the risks of lending my vehicle to someone who might drive under the influence. His response shattered me: "F*ck you, B**ch! I hope you die in here!" He stormed out, leaving me in tears, grappling with the magnitude of his cruelty.

That day marked a profound shift within me, eroding my ability to trust. The pain of his words and the sense of betrayal felt insurmountable, and I realized that I would carry scars from that moment forward. Even now, I continue to navigate those trust issues in therapy.

Yearning for a life partner who could love me through my challenges, I embarked on another relationship with a man I met through a mutual friend. He was charming and mature, treating me with respect and thoughtfulness. He was employed, owned a car, and had his own home. After six months of dating, he invited me to Thanksgiving dinner with his family, and I embraced the opportunity, feeling welcomed and appreciated.

As I underwent dialysis treatments, he often sat with me, bringing food and snacks to ease my discomfort during the four-hour sessions. We made plans for dinner after one of my treatments, but less than a minute after he left, I received a text that shattered the afterglow of his visit: "Hey, Mrs. (his last name). What would you like to eat for dinner?" I stared at the phone for a very long time trying to make sense of what I was reading, even though it was a very clear message. My heart raced with disbelief. He was married? How could he be? We had shared Thanksgiving Day together, and he had been so attentive. A whirlwind of emotions swept over me as I sat in that dialysis chair—shock, hurt, anger, and betrayal—leading to tears as the familiar ache of deception washed over me.

”

These experiences have left their mark on my heart, mind, and spirit, but just as cocoa butter soothes scars, the diligent work that therapy requires for success helps those marks fade over time.

In a determined attempt to handle the situation with dignity, I devised a plan. After my treatment, I drove home and locked my driveway gate and ignored his calls and texts. When he arrived, he knocked frantically at my door, pleading for an opportunity to explain. I stood firm, threatening to call the police if he didn't leave, and he left immediately.

In the weeks that followed, I grieved deeply. Part of that process involved discarding every gift he had given me, including a beautiful sundress from his sister's boutique. I decided to meet her to return the dress. I told her about the breakup and asked her opinion on why he invited me to Thanksgiving dinner if he was married. It was then that I learned that the family believed I was aware of his marital status and was okay with it. I was left speechless, grappling with the painful reality that this man had misrepresented our relationship to his family.

The strong desire for companionship led me to repeat patterns. I found myself dating yet another man—tall, charming, and handsome, yet again living with his mother and often unemployed. This time, I later realized he saw me as a potential source of financial support, mistakenly thinking my chronic illness qualified me for government assistance.

Reflecting on these five years post-diagnosis, I realize that my self-esteem and fear of mortality shaped my choices then. My longing for love led me to lower my standards, allowing unhealthy relationships to flourish. Yet, I am grateful for God's strength that carried me through those times and for the healing power of therapy. These experiences have left their mark on my heart, mind, and spirit, but just as cocoa butter soothes scars, the diligent work that therapy requires for success helps those marks fade over time.

Living with chronic health issues often alters the dating landscape. We contend with questions of desirability, fearing that our condition may render us burdensome. Our fear of morality becomes intertwined with what appears as love, and we worry about the fleeting nature of both. In my haste to find a partner, I compromised my standards, failed to vet potential partners thoroughly, and accepted unacceptable behaviors.

Through these situations, I learned the importance of resilience and the value of self-love. While the journey may be filled with challenges, I now understand that my worth is not defined by my circumstances but by the strength I carry within.

Not only so, but we also glory in our sufferings, because we know that suffering produces perseverance; perseverance, character; and character, hope.

-Romans 5:3-4

Let's Chat About It:
Resilient Heart

1. Have health challenges influenced your approach to relationships and dating?
2. What roles do self-esteem and fear of mortality play in my relationship choices? Can you relate to this in your own life?
3. I mention how therapy has helped me heal emotionally. How important do you think therapy is in overcoming past traumas, especially those related to relationships?
4. What are your thoughts on my decision to set boundaries with men who were unavailable or untrustworthy? How would you have handled those situations?
5. How do you think chronic health conditions impact romantic relationships in general?
6. How does the scripture from Romans 5:3-4 ("suffering produces perseverance; perseverance, character; and character, hope") apply to my experiences in this chapter?
7. What does the metaphor of "applying cocoa butter to scars" mean to you in the context of emotional healing? Do you have a similar personal metaphor for healing?
8. If you were to offer advice to me based on my experiences in this chapter, what would it be?

Did anything in this chapter inspire you? Let me know by leaving a review on Amazon—I'd love to read it.

8.
Faith Refined

When I began dialysis, I was utterly overwhelmed, both emotionally and physically. Fear for my life clouded my every thought, and my self-esteem plunged. The social worker at the dialysis center was such a lifeline. She walked me through the next steps, helping me sign up for Medicare, explaining that it was a requirement for all dialysis patients, and reassuring me that coverage would begin after my transplant.

But even her support couldn't shake the despair I felt in those early days. As I sat in that dialysis chair, I was frequently told by staff and other patients, "You're too young and beautiful to be here." I'd smile weakly in agreement, but their words challenged my own disbelief. There was a patient at the center even younger than me—just 18 years old. Seeing her there broke my heart. Here I was, feeling robbed of my vitality, and she hadn't even had a chance to really live her life yet.

I was a woman building my faith, but during those early treatments, my faith was nowhere to be found. The nurses would connect me to the dialysis machine, speaking encouragement over me: "You don't belong here. God is going to heal you." But in my heart, I doubted every word. The fear was too loud, drowning out any possibility of hope.

My family, friends, co-workers, and church family never stopped believing. They prayed for my healing when I didn't have the strength or faith to pray for myself. They really stood in the gap with big faith on my behalf. Their faith carried me.

Slowly, ever so slowly, my faith became reignited. Over time, I found myself speaking words of hope again. When people asked about the bandages on my arm, I'd say, "I'm on dialysis, but God is going to heal me." And when they asked how, I'd confidently reply, "I don't know, but I know He will."

While adjusting to a low-sodium diet—one of many hurdles in this journey—my social worker helped me start the process of being placed on the kidney transplant wait list. If you're like I was back then, you might assume that needing dialysis treatments automatically puts a person on the transplant wait list. But it doesn't. Before someone can be added, they have to prove that they are otherwise healthy, with no conditions that could compromise the transplant's success.

I was handed a list of 31 tests I needed to complete in order to be added to the wait list. And so began a long process—contacting specialists, setting appointments, waiting for appointment dates, undergoing tests, waiting for results, and reporting back to my social worker and dialysis center. It felt like an endless loop of doctors, waiting rooms, and medical jargon.

If you take away nothing else from my story, let it be this: if you can, accompany someone you care about to their medical appointments. Sitting with them, chatting to take their mind off things, simply being present—it all makes a world of difference. Your presence can remind someone that their life matters, that they are loved, and that they are worth fighting for. Your support can encourage them to feel better and it can motivate them to do all they can to fight for better health.

After countless appointments, I began to wish I had someone with me. Every waiting room started to look the same, with numbing boredom and palpable loneliness. I'd watch other patients surrounded by loved ones—spouses, siblings, friends—while I sat alone. It made me happy that they had support for what they were battling, someone who took the time out of their schedule, their lives, maybe even took time off of work, to come and wait with them. But it also made me sad that I didn't have that. My parents were retired and lived in another state, the man I was dating didn't show up for me, and my extended family and friends didn't fully understand what I was going through. So, to make myself feel better as I sat by myself, I'd whisper, "Well, it's just You and me, God." Perhaps He wanted it that way. Perhaps He needed me to know that it was the two of us—just He and I—getting through this together.

It took a year to complete all 31 tests, a year where my physical isolation mirrored a deep emotional struggle. I spiraled into a depression. I didn't enjoy going to work. My romantic relationships crumbled. I grew frustrated with my dietary restrictions to the point that I stopped eating altogether. My weight dropped to a frail 95 pounds. I was shrinking, physically and emotionally, and no one seemed to notice.

Accompany someone you care about to their medical appointments. Sitting with them, chatting to take their mind off things, simply being present—it all makes a world of difference. Your presence can remind someone that their life matters, that they are loved, and that they are worth fighting for.

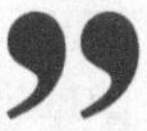

One day, I lay on the couch, weak and exhausted, thinking about how easy it would be to just close my eyes and never wake up. The thought felt like a strange relief. In that moment, God reminded me of something from my past. He brought to mind my high school teacher, Nancy Erdvig, who had once driven me from Miami to Orlando (a four-hour drive) for a Future Business Leaders of America conference, as I served as State President that year. Mrs. Erdvig, the FBLA Sponsor, had sacrificed a weekend with her own family to take me. God said, "Think about all the time, effort, and love people have poured into you—your teachers, your parents. You can't give up now. You can't let their sacrifices be in vain."

The thought of disappointing them, of throwing away the love and support I'd been given, brought me to tears. I realized that I couldn't give up. Not on them, not on myself.

I started making small changes. I signed up for a meal delivery service, though the food was awful. I joined a gym, even though I didn't go as often as I should have. But just the act of showing up those few times gave me a spark of motivation. Slowly, I began to eat again. I regained control of my diet. Although the financial burden of constant doctor's appointments, co-pays, and medicine weighed heavily on me, I managed to push through.

That year was one of the hardest of my life. But it taught me that resilience is not just about bouncing back—it's about finding the strength to move forward, even when every part of you wants to quit.

But those who hope in the Lord will renew their strength. They will soar on wings like eagles; they will run and not grow weary; they will walk and not be faint.

-Isaiah 40:31

Let's Chat About It:
Faith Refined

1. How did my journey through dialysis challenge or affirm your own understanding of resilience?
2. Faith played a major role in my healing process. How did you interpret the moments when I struggled with faith, and how did those moments contribute to my growth?
3. The theme of support is present throughout the chapter, with friends, family, and coworkers standing in the gap for me. Have you ever had someone stand in the gap for you during a difficult time? What impact did that have on you?
4. What do you think I meant by saying, "Resilience is not just about bouncing back—it's about finding the strength to move forward"? How does this definition of resilience compare to your own?
5. My journey included a series of medical tests and waiting periods. How did these moments of waiting shape my understanding of patience and perseverance?
6. How does the scripture Isaiah 40:31 resonate with my experiences in this chapter? Can you think of a time in your life when this scripture held true for you?
7. Loneliness is a recurring theme in this chapter. What strategies for coping with loneliness have helped you?

If you connected with something in this chapter, I'd appreciate hearing your thoughts. Please leave a review on Amazon.

9.
Beauty Beyond the Battle

The summer of 2008 marked a significant milestone—ten years since my high school graduation. A reunion was on the horizon, a time typically filled with excitement as people gather to relive memories and share their experiences over the past ten years. It was a moment to highlight career achievements, family growth, and personal adventures. However, for me, the thought of attending the reunion was bittersweet.

On one hand, I looked forward to seeing old friends and hearing their stories. On the other, I couldn't ignore the nagging concern about how I would be perceived. I was nervous about what people may think once they saw the huge bandage on my chest covering the chest catheter, the darker skin (a common side effect of dialysis treatments), and the thick tan gauze that is wrapped around my arm after dialysis treatments. When the organizers asked me to present an award as part of the weekend of events, I hesitated. Normally, I would have jumped at the chance. This time, I wondered if I was ready to stand in front of everyone in such a vulnerable state.

I chose to attend. I realized that this reunion was a once-in-a-lifetime experience. I refused to let my insecurities rob me of that.

To my surprise, the weekend was more fulfilling than I could have imagined. It was wonderful seeing how my classmates had blossomed into their adult lives—sharing their families, careers, and unique paths. There were endless laughs, stories, and memories relived. Sure, some people noticed my arm and asked about it, but when I shared my story, the response was heartwarming. Instead of judgment, there was empathy. People prayed for me, asked how they could help me, and some even asked how they could become organ donors themselves. That reunion was one of the first moments I realized that my story had power. It could be a tool for raising awareness and for inspiring others to become organ, eye, and tissue donors. My health journey was no longer something to hide but something to share.

If you would like to make a difference in someone's life by giving them a second chance, please go to https://register.donatelifecalifornia.org/somonesstory and register today.

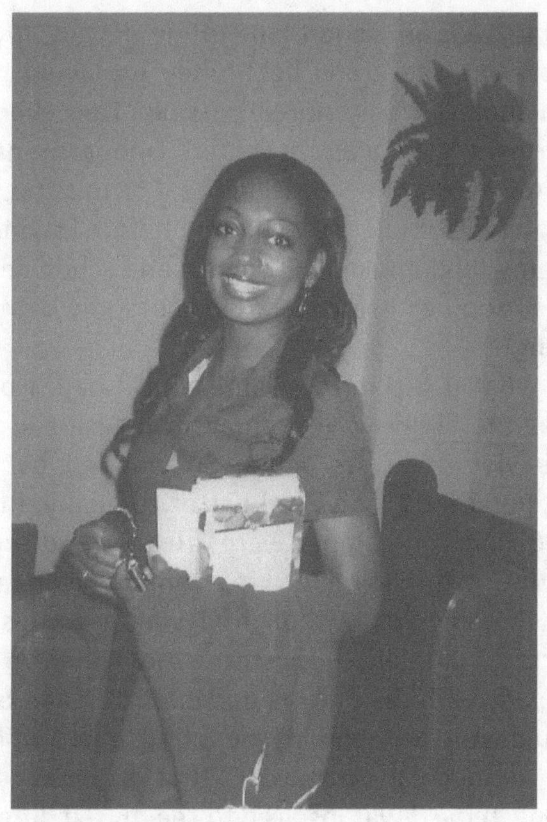

10 Year High School Class Reunion Sunday Service

The following year, a high school friend, James McGriff, invited me on a trip to Jamaica. He was a finalist in a modeling contest, and the prize was an all-expense-paid trip to compete in the finals. He could bring along one guest, and without hesitation, I said yes. All I needed was a plane ticket, and everything else was covered. It was an easy decision.

The trip was scheduled for April 30th through May 3rd, 2009, and I was still on dialysis. I wasn't sure if international travel was even an option, but to my delight, my dialysis team gave me the green light. They explained that with proper planning, it was entirely possible. They even told me about cruises with dialysis centers onboard—news that opened my eyes to new possibilities. For this trip, the plan was simple: I'd complete a treatment before leaving, closely monitor my fluid intake while away, and schedule another session as soon as I returned. I was ecstatic. Jamaica was happening!

And what a trip it was. James and I had a blast! We stayed at the all-inclusive Hedonism II resort in Negril, a place as vibrant as its name. Surrounded by stunning scenery, good food, and even better company, I felt alive. The modeling contestants were friendly and welcoming towards me, even though I wasn't competing. In fact, some of the women initially thought I was a contestant—an unexpected confidence booster. Who would've thought that the lady with the dialysis-darkened skin and bandaged arm could still be seen as beautiful even while going through a medical endeavor? That experience shifted something in me. I was inspired to see myself differently.

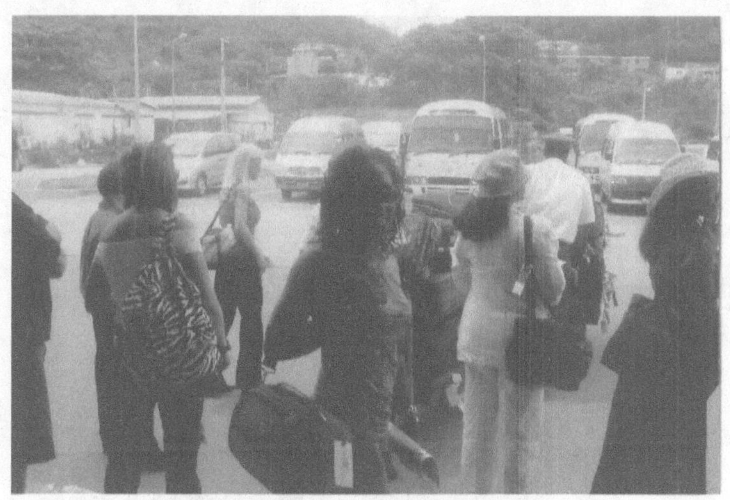

Arriving at the airport in Jamaica 2009

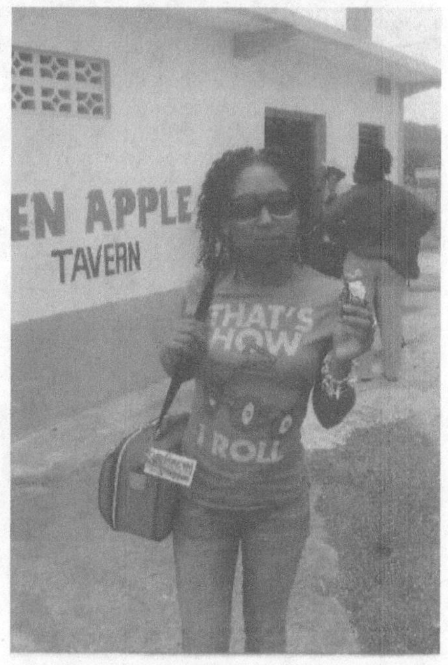

Making a stop for snacks on the way to Negril

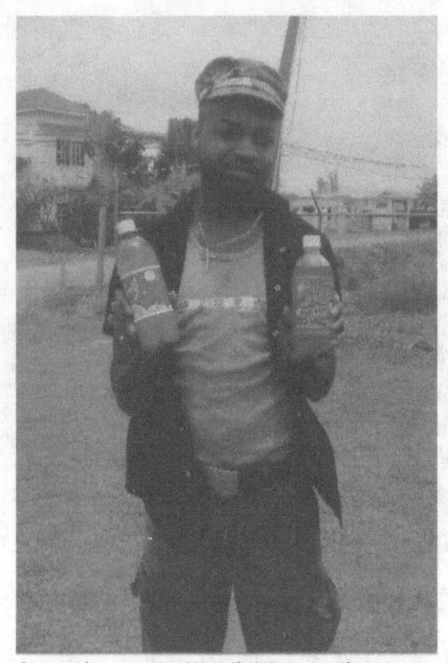

Making a stop for snacks on the way to Negril. Hi, James!

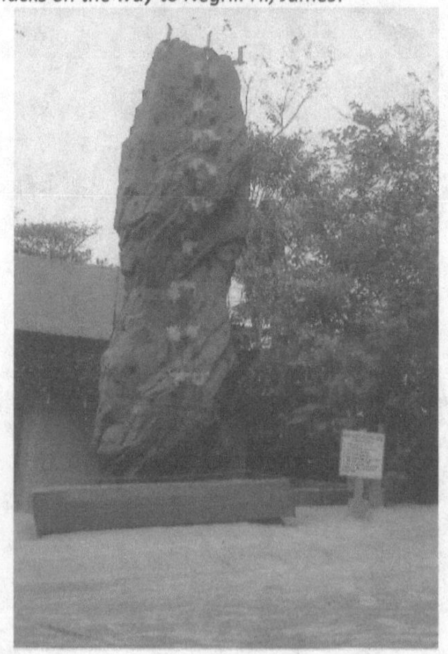

Hedonism II 2009

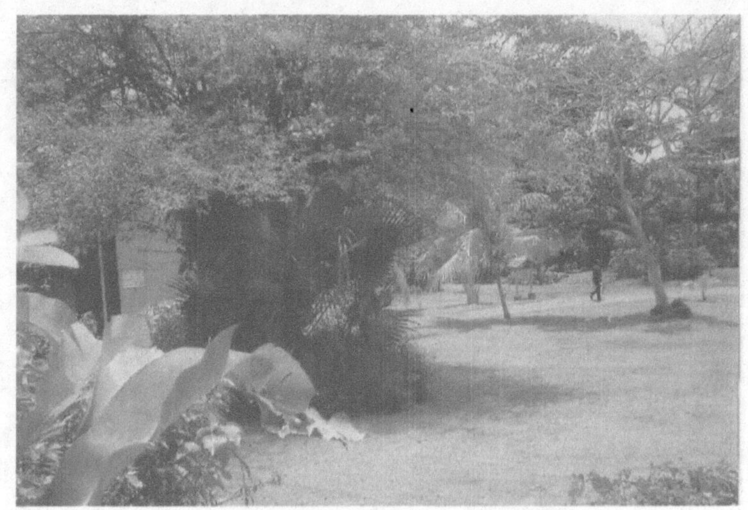

Hedonism II 2009

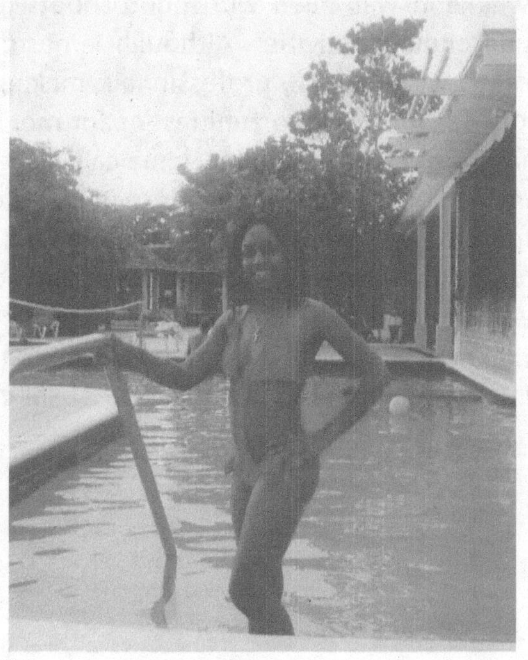

Hedonism II 2009

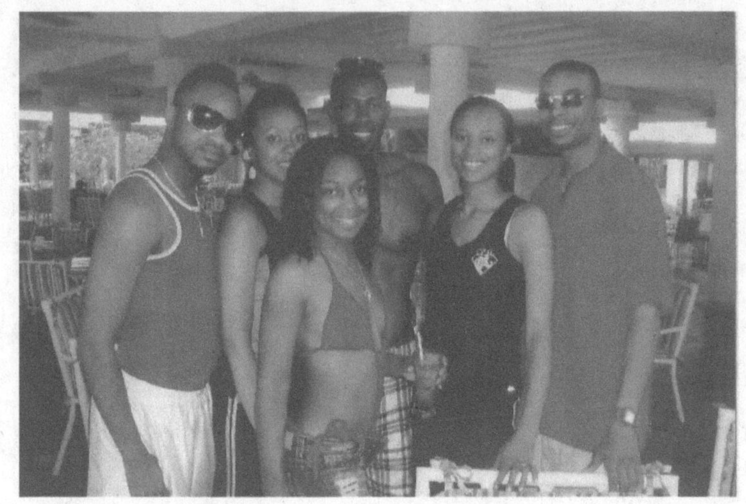

The model contestants and me

The weekend was filled with photoshoots, beachside parties, and endless activities. Although James didn't win, he networked with industry professionals, making valuable connections for future opportunities. As for me, I indulged in the island's delights, including Jamaica's signature rum cream, and let loose, enjoying every second. I even got so caught up in the fun that I didn't watch my fluid intake as carefully as I should have. When I returned and stepped on the scale at my next dialysis treatment, the numbers told the story. I knew I'd pay for it in cramps during the session, and I did. It was painful, but in my mind—absolutely worth it.

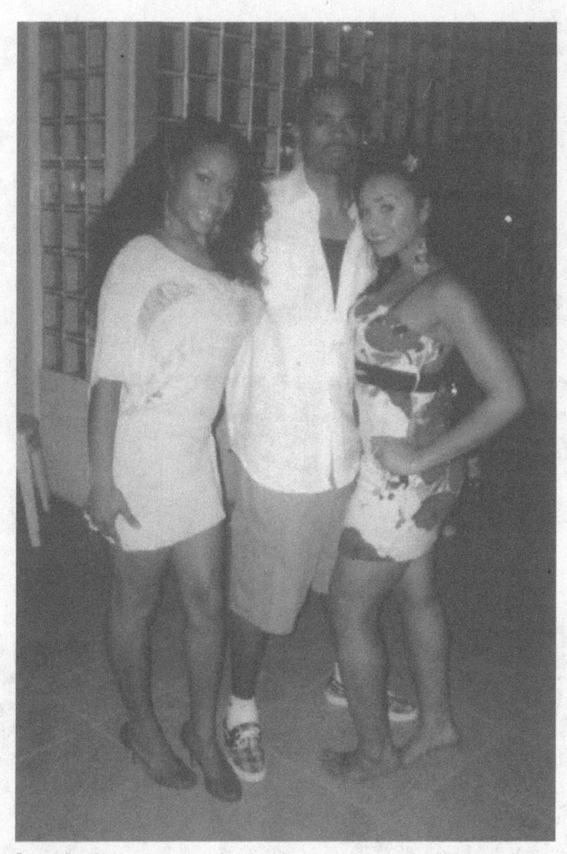

Model Contest Organizers

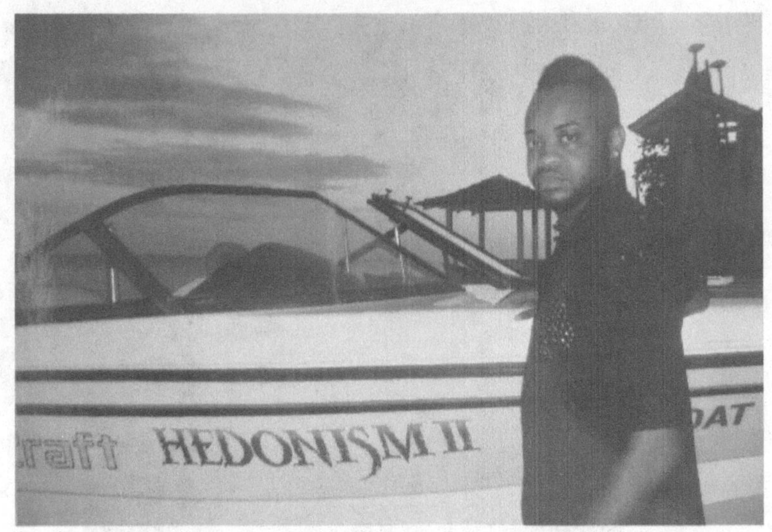

James

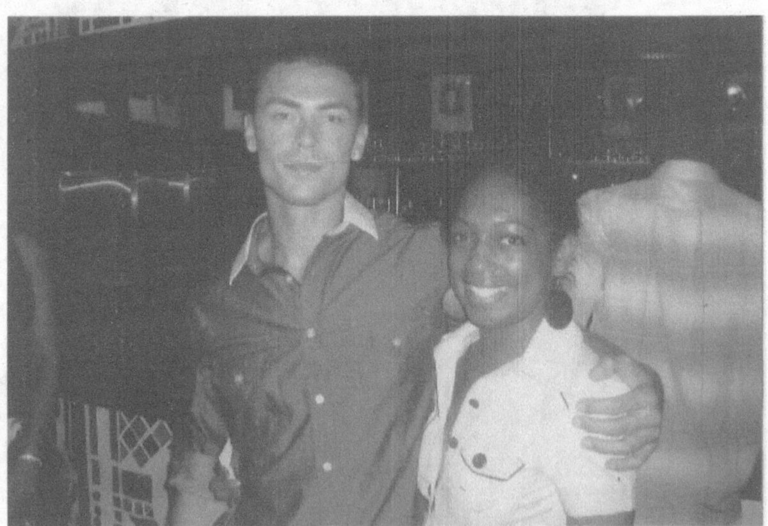
Me posing with the winner of the modeling contest

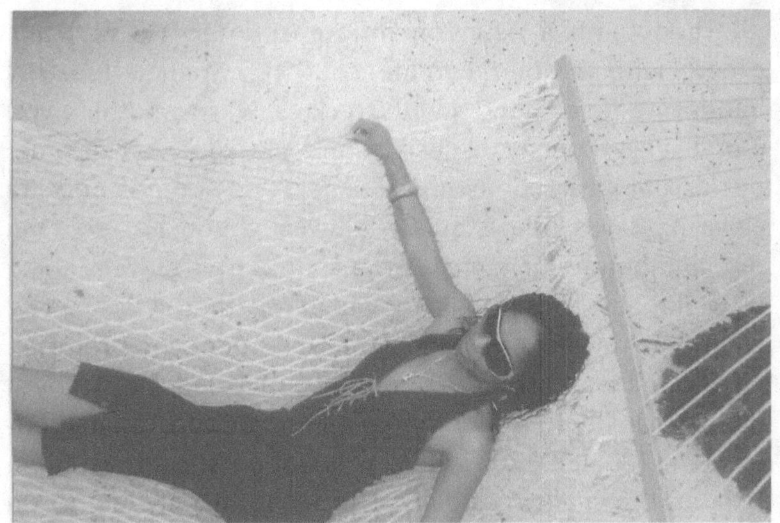

Enjoying the amenities at Hedonism II

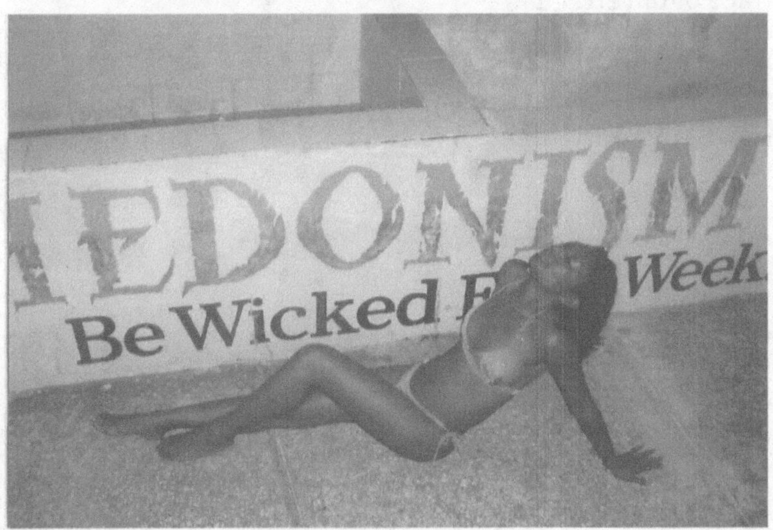

Being around the models all weekend started rubbing off on me

Then came a new romantic encounter. He was tall, broad, with a quiet confidence that intrigued me. His handsome face, marked with freckles, was something you didn't see every day, especially on a Black man. Over time, our casual interactions grew longer, and soon, it became clear that I was interested. Once he caught on, he asked me out, and before long, we were a couple. Things were going so well that we eventually moved in together. It was a new chapter in my life, one filled with excitement and promise.

From a high school reunion that revealed the strength of vulnerability to a spontaneous trip that boosted my self-esteem, 2008 and 2009 were years of personal revelation. Despite the challenges dialysis brought into my life, those experiences taught me the beauty of sharing my story, embracing new opportunities, and finding joy even in the face of uncertainty.

That class reunion was one of the first moments I realized my story had power. It could be a tool for raising awareness and for inspiring others to become organ, eye, and tissue donors. My health journey was no longer something to hide but something to share.

Praise be to the God and Father of our Lord Jesus Christ, the Father of compassion and the God of all comfort, who comforts us in all our troubles, so that we can comfort those in any trouble...

-2 Corinthians 1:3-4

Let's Chat About It: Beauty Beyond the Battle

1. How did my experiences at the reunion resonate with your own experiences of reconnecting with old friends? Have you ever felt vulnerable in similar situations?
2. I mention realizing the power of sharing my story. Why do you think sharing personal experiences can be transformative for both the storyteller and the listeners?
3. How did my interactions with my classmates evolve during the reunion? What role do you think empathy played in their responses to my health journey?
4. How do you think chronic health issues influence a person's sense of self? Did my journey change your perception of how health challenges can shape relationships?
5. How do you think societal perceptions of health and beauty impact individuals dealing with medical conditions? Did my experience challenge any stereotypes you may hold?
6. After reading this chapter, what actions or changes do you feel inspired to take in your own life or community? How can we support others who are navigating similar challenges?

Did this chapter touch you in a meaningful way? I'd love to hear your reflections—feel free to leave a review on Amazon.

10.
The Weight of Waiting

In September 2009, a letter arrived that would alter the trajectory of my life. It confirmed my placement on the kidney transplant waitlist in Miami, Florida. Overjoyed, I braced myself for what I thought would be a long wait at the bottom of a list exceeding 7,000 people. However, I soon learned that the process depended on a complex web of factors—blood type, tissue compatibility, and the availability of a matching organ in my vicinity. The wait would be unpredictable, but at last, I had a glimmer of hope that my life could soon return to normal... or so I thought.

On Thanksgiving night, November 26, 2009, my phone rang after dinner, igniting a surge of anticipation. The hospital informed me of a potential kidney match. Ecstatic, I raced to Jackson Memorial Hospital, where a friendly nurse greeted me and guided me through the process which included a blood draw. Afterward, I returned home to await the results—a nerve-wracking wait that felt like an eternity, my body taut with uneasiness as I held my breath, hoping for the best. I was told that the call could come up to eight hours after the blood draw, or more. So, I waited.

The call finally came. "There was someone else who was a closer match this time. I'm so sorry." Devastation washed over me. I couldn't fully process in that moment that receiving a call that day meant someone else had just lost a loved one. For their family, Thanksgiving Day would never be the same.

A couple of months later, while attending a conference in Fort Lauderdale, FL, I received another call from the hospital. Dropping everything, I sped as I drove the thirty minutes to Miami, greeted once again by that same kind nurse. After the blood draw, I returned home, my heart racing with hope. Yet, eight hours later, I received the same disappointing news: "Not this time, Ms. Washington."

With each call, I learned more about the process. Each time I was contacted, several other patients that were a close matched were summoned to the hospital for blood analysis, and the closest match would be determined among us. After my third call, I had grown weary of the routine. This time, I waited, checking my watch as the hours slipped by without a call. Finally, I took the initiative and called the hospital myself. The news was unchanged: it wasn't my time yet.

By the fourth call, I had become somewhat of a regular visitor to the lab. I recognized the phlebotomist and made light of my situation, saying, "Okay, thank you. See you next time!" Her stern response, "No, you won't!" caught me off guard. It was her way of expressing confidence that this would be my match, a small beacon of hope amidst my growing cynicism. The outcome was the same: I wasn't the chosen one. In time, I learned that my frequent calls were a sign of my position near the top of the waitlist.

Soon, I began to visualize what life after a transplant might look like. As I pondered my future, I realized the necessity of preparing my work environment for the reality of living with a compromised immune system post-transplant. At the time, I was an elementary school teacher—a role filled with seasonal colds passed around by eager little hands. It dawned on me that I would need a clean, controlled space to mitigate exposure to germs.

I proactively submitted a Family Medical Leave Act (FMLA) request for accommodations post-surgery. I sought a classroom equipped with its own bathroom to minimize interactions with communal restrooms and asked for more frequent cleaning of this space. I felt positive, knowing that allowing plenty of time for an approval would help me be better prepared for when the time finally came.

To my shock, my principal rejected my request outright. Instinctively, I recognized that this battle would require reinforcements. I reached out to the school district's Americans with Disabilities (ADA) office, sharing my experience with a representative who was appalled by the principal's response. "This is a straightforward request for a legitimate reason," she asserted, promising to advocate on my behalf.

Weeks passed, and eventually, I received news from the ADA office: my request had been approved. The representative revealed that my principal had initially resisted but conceded once the legal implications of her decision were clarified. "I can't believe she actually tried to fight us on this!" she exclaimed.

In June 2010, the school district faced a surplus of teachers, leading to potential furloughs for those hired last. Frustrated by my principal's treatment, I considered taking personal leave to step away from an environment that felt hostile to my well-being. Yet, my request was again denied. I realized I had one more option: I could apply for medical leave due to my ongoing dialysis treatments.

”

...expand your network, stay informed about your rights, and use your voice. Advocating for yourself can be daunting, but it is essential, especially when facing challenges that impact your health and well-being.

Submitting my medical leave request felt liberating. It was an undeniable necessity, and my short- and long-term disability insurance would cover most of my salary during my absence.

Reflecting on this chapter of my life, I recognize it as a pivotal lesson in self-advocacy. Had I not fought for necessary accommodations or sought support from resources beyond my immediate environment, my health would have been at risk in a workplace fraught with potential dangers. Let my experience serve as a reminder to expand your network, stay informed about your rights, and use your voice. Advocating for yourself can be daunting, but it is essential, especially when facing challenges that impact your health and well-being. This is easier said than done at times and it can be scary to do, especially depending on who or what you may be up against and what you stand to lose but do it anyway. You have a voice and rights for the reason of using them at the most appropriate times.

By September 2010, I had been on the kidney transplant waitlist for over a year. The cycle of tests and appointments loomed ahead of me, each year requiring a renewal of evaluations to maintain my place on the list. Initially, the news felt discouraging, yet I mustered up my strength and began the process anew, determined to persevere through whatever lay ahead.

But if we hope for what we do not yet have, we wait for it patiently.

-Romans 8:25

Let's Chat About It:
The Weight of Waiting

1. How did my experiences with the kidney transplant waitlist resonate with your own experiences of waiting or facing uncertainty in life?
2. What are some ways I demonstrated self-advocacy, and how can you apply this in your own lives when facing challenges?
3. In what ways did I display resilience throughout my journey? Can you think of a time when you had to be resilient in your own life?
4. How important was the support from the ADA representative and the phlebotomist in my journey? What role do support systems play in your own challenges?
5. How did faith influence my journey? How does spirituality or faith play a role in your own life during difficult times?
6. What challenges did I face in my work environment, and how did those challenges affect my health? What steps can workplaces take to better support employees with health concerns?
7. What insights does this chapter provide about the psychological aspects of waiting for a life-changing event?

If this chapter spoke to you, I'd love for you to share your thoughts in an Amazon review.

11.
Midnight Miracles

One evening in mid-November, I settled onto my couch, the glow of the television casting a warm light in the dim room. I was watching the movie, *For Colored Girls*; the haunting narrative gripping my attention. As the clock ticked closer to 9:00 pm, I found myself riveted to a particularly harrowing scene. The character Beau, played by Michael Ealy, was in the throes of a drunken rage, dangling his two young children from a high-rise apartment window while their mother, Crystal (Kimberly Elise), desperately pleaded with him to stop.

"No way he's going to let go," I thought, reassuring myself that movies don't usually portray such evil acts against children. But then, it happened—he actually released their tiny arms. I could hear their terrified screams echo in my mind as they fell, the horrifying thud resonating with a visceral intensity that left me speechless. Devastation washed over me; tears streamed down my face as I wrestled with the rawness of that moment. It felt too real.

As I was lost in my emotions, the phone rang, jolting me from my trance. I recognized the number—one I had seen several times that day, during my restless wait for news. "Hello?" I answered, still shaken from the film. I braced myself for the familiar letdown: "I'm sorry, Ms. Washington. Unfortunately, you were not a match this time."

Instead, the voice on the other end of the phone delivered life-changing news: "Ms. Washington, we have a kidney for you. You need to report to the emergency room by midnight tonight."

Suddenly, I felt light-headed, the words swirling in a chaotic rush that drowned out everything else. Grabbing a notepad, I hastily scribbled down instructions, thanking the caller profusely before she hung up. I stood there, a whirlwind of emotions surging through me, unsure of what to do next.

Desperate to share my news, I called my parents' home phone and their cell phones—no answers. I left a voicemail, my heart sinking. Next, I dialed my boyfriend, Chip, who was at work. I needed a ride to the hospital, as the instructions required. He assured me he was on his way. I reached out to friends and family, but the irony struck me hard; not a single person was available at this crucial moment. Frustrated, I updated my voicemail greeting to inform callers of my situation and posted an update on Facebook.

Realizing I needed to prepare, I began packing a bag. Although I was advised during the transplant orientation class to have one ready, I had neglected to do so. I quickly threw in a few outfits and essentials, wanting to be ready to go when Chip arrived. With only two hours to get to Jackson Memorial Hospital in downtown Miami, time was of the essence.

A tumultuous kaleidoscope of emotions swirled within me. I felt the weight of the film's impact lingering as I tried to reconcile the gravity of my situation. Why was Chip taking so long? Was I ready for this monumental change? I prayed for a smooth surgery and pondered what life would be like post-transplant.

Then, the phone rang again. My heart raced, hopeful it might be my mom or Chip. But it was my dialysis nurse. She mentioned an earlier dialysis appointment had opened up for the next day, but I could hardly focus on that— "I just got called for my transplant!" I exclaimed. "That's why I have an open appointment," she said. "Someone else got called tonight, too! Maybe you'll meet her!" That was a bright note amid the chaos.

When Chip finally arrived, he apologized for the delay, explaining his boss had been difficult about him leaving work. "But it's an emergency!" I protested. "I know, he's a jerk," he replied. I felt guilty for causing an issue for him, especially when he later shared that he'd received a write-up for leaving.

We made it to the emergency room just in time. Sadly, Chip had to return to work, leaving me alone once more—a familiar feeling on this journey.

As I checked in, a woman entered the room and announced that she was there for a transplant as she checked-in at the station next to me. I felt a surge of excitement; when I asked about her dialysis facility, she confirmed it was South Broward DaVita. She mentioned my dialysis nurse's name, and we were both stunned by the coincidence. We had shared the same treatment space but had never met—our schedules had never aligned. As it turned out, we shared the same blood and tissue type. Much later we discovered that we received our transplants from the same donor.

"We have a kidney for you. We need you to report to the emergency room by midnight tonight."

We continued to chat as we completed our paperwork. Once I finished, I was escorted to the surgery prep area, exchanging wishes of good luck with my new acquaintance.

By 2:00 am, I lay on a gurney in the operating room. Nurses and anesthesiologists introduced themselves, their calm demeanors easing my nerves. "Everything will be fine," one reassured me. I smiled and whispered my gratitude. That was the last thing I remembered.

I awoke, surrounded by a maze of tubes, my body heavy and restrained. The first face I saw was my mother's, worry etched into her features, while my dad sat beside her, equally concerned. "Hi baby, how are you feeling?" my mom asked. "Hi, Mom! You got here fast!" I replied, bewildered. "We've been driving all night," she said, her voice thick with emotion.

The strain of the night caught up with my mom, and in a moment of overwhelm, she fainted. Panic surged through me. I cried out, unsure of what was happening. The nurse told me that I had to calm down because my body could not endure any stress right after surgery. My dad was there to catch her before she fell to the ground as my mother's condition drew attention. Nurses quickly surrounded her, waving papers to fan her, bringing her back to consciousness. "I'm fine," she insisted, though I wasn't convinced. After a tense moment, my dad headed to the cafeteria to get her something to eat, and I was moved to a recovery room. On the other side of the curtain was Dion, the woman I'd met earlier. We exchanged smiles, our paths finally converging.

The next morning, I awoke to a precise, assertive nurse, who dropped a massive bag filled with bottles of medication on the table beside my bed. "You'll need to figure out your medication regimen," she explained, and I stared at her in disbelief. "I just had surgery yesterday! How can I manage this?" She handed me a workbook, explaining that it was to help keep track of everything, and then she left me to navigate this immense task on my own.

Overwhelmed, I glanced at Dion, who shared my incredulity. We shook our heads at the absurdity of it all. I reasoned that if I messed up my medication, it was better to do it under watchful eyes in a hospital rather than at home. At least I wouldn't be bored during recovery.

A few moments later, my mom returned from getting coffee, her eyes widening as she took in the scene. "What's all this?" she asked, stunned at the array of bottles. I explained, and together, we attempted to make sense of the chaos.

Doctors made their rounds, asking about my recovery. I expressed my feelings of overwhelm, receiving shallow assurances in response.

After only six days post-transplant, I was discharged from the hospital. This was a lot faster than I imagined, yet I was ready. Dion would remain in the hospital for a while longer due to complications, and my heart ached for her.

As I prepared to leave, I reflected on the journey: I received a second chance at life through kidney transplantation on November 18, 2010. 769 days, 14 hours, and 27 minutes had passed from my first dialysis treatment to this moment. I was heading home to start a new chapter of my life.

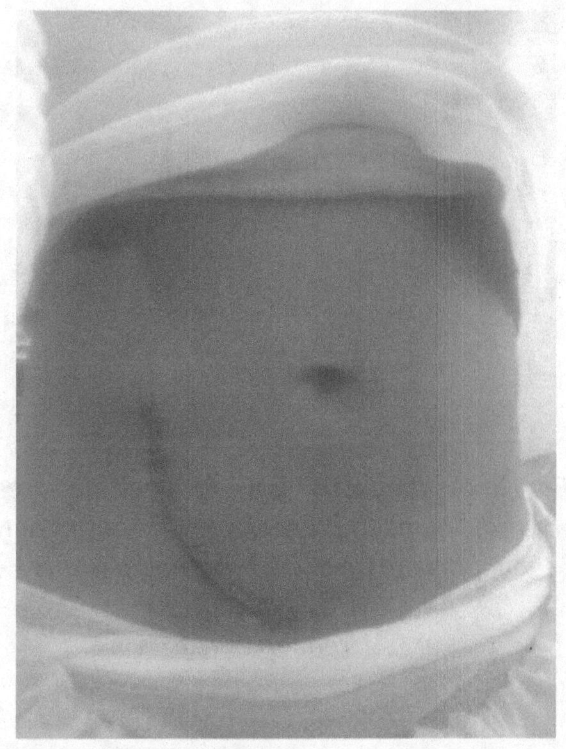

The scar from my kidney transplant days after surgery.

For I know the plans I have for you," declares the Lord, "plans to prosper you and not to harm you, plans to give you hope and a future.

-Jeremiah 29:11

Let's Chat About It:
Midnight Miracles

1. What emotions did you experience while reading about the moment I received the call for the transplant?
2. How does the juxtaposition of watching a powerful movie scene and receiving life-changing news reflect the unpredictability of life?
3. In what ways does the chapter explore the theme of hope amidst uncertainty, and how can that apply to our own lives?
4. What significance do you find in the connection between me and the woman I meet at the hospital, and how does it reflect the shared human experience?
5. What insights do you gain from the dialogue between me and the medical staff regarding the responsibility of managing health post-surgery?
6. Have you watched the movie, *For Colored Girls*? If so, what are your thoughts on the scene described in this chapter?
7. What has been your favorite chapter in the book so far? Why?
8. What questions would you ask me about anything that you've read so far?

Did this chapter resonate with you? I'd love to hear what you think—leave a review on Amazon and let me know

12.
The Gift

Returning to my childhood home in Miami felt like stepping into a time capsule. I stayed in the bedroom where I had once dreamt as a young girl, but now, as an adult, it felt different—smaller somehow, as if the room had shrunk over the years. My parents were my pillars of strength during this time. My mother, meticulous as ever, ensured that my sutures were cleaned several times a day and she was on top of my medication regimen. She gently helped me dress and assisted me in taking small walks around the house, mindful of the sharp pain from the vertical incision near my navel. Each step was a challenge, but with her by my side, I felt cared for and safe.

My father, ever the provider, took charge of the kitchen, creating low-sodium meals that met my new dietary restrictions. His presence brought a sense of calm, proactively handling tasks that needed doing without complaint. Together, they embodied love in its purest form, helping me through the long, slow process of recovery.

The homecare nurse sent by the post-transplant team at the hospital initially visited three times a week. After the second week, however, he admitted that there was little left for him to do. My vitals were stable, my mother had bathing under control, and my father handled meals with precision. His job had already been done by my parents. The routine doctor appointments, though, were non-negotiable—three times a week, like clockwork. My mother drove me to each one, as I wasn't yet cleared to drive, still under the effects of pain and an array of medications.

When my father had to return to Georgia to manage my parents' affairs, it marked the first time they had spent time apart in their 40 years of marriage. It pained me to think that my recovery had caused such a separation, even if just for a while. Yet, I knew it was necessary.

The first outing beyond the hospital circuit was Christmas shopping with my mom. We only made it to two stores before exhaustion overtook me. My stamina was still low, but there was progress. By January, I was strong enough to transition to my new apartment in Hollywood, and with my mother's help, I got settled into my new space. Each day brought more progress, and by February, I was itching to re-engage with the world. Though I wasn't yet cleared to return to work, I found fulfillment volunteering at the Miami-Dade County Public Schools administrative offices, working alongside a fellow sorority sister.

As the summer ended and a new school year began, I returned to work, this time at North Miami Senior High School. High school offered a unique environment, and it turned out to be a perfect fit for me, especially with my compromised immune system. Older students presented fewer health risk exposures for me compared to the little ones in elementary school. I thrived there. Those high school students reinvigorated my passion for teaching, and the sense of purpose that came with it made this period the most rewarding of my career.

Physically, I was in great health—no complications, no setbacks, just pure gratitude for the second chance I'd been given. My medication regimen had been reduced from twenty different types of pills to just two: Myfortic and Prograf, which are immune suppressant meds that I will have to take from now on. Life had returned to a beautiful rhythm, and I marveled at the blessing that was my kidney transplant.

During this time, I stayed close with Dion, my "kidney sister." She worked in financial services, and January through April was her busiest season, offering tax preparation services. She returned to work much earlier than advised, just under two months post-surgery, driven by the demands of her job. Unfortunately, the stress and physical exertion led to complications with her kidney function, and she found herself back in the hospital. The scare was enough for her to step back and focus on her recovery, understanding the importance of pacing herself.

The source of my gift—an 18-year-old young man who lost his life to gun violence—was never far from my thoughts. His family, in the midst of their unimaginable grief, made the selfless decision to donate his organs, allowing him to live on through others, including me. The hospital gave me the opportunity to write a letter to his family, a task that weighed heavily on my heart. How do I even begin to express gratitude for such an unimaginable sacrifice? I wrestled with finding the right balance—conveying deep appreciation for my renewed life and being sensitive to their profound loss.

Eventually, I found the words, but it took time. I wrote the letter, not just with my hand but with my heart, offering them my highest thanks. It was important to me that they knew their loved one had not only saved my life but many others as well.

”

How do I even begin to express gratitude for such an unimaginable sacrifice? I wrestled with finding the right balance—not wanting to celebrate my renewed life too much, while being sensitive to their profound loss.

His legacy continues in me, and I hope that knowledge provided some measure of comfort to his family.

For the rest of my life, I will carry that young man's spirit within me, honoring the great gift he and his family bestowed upon me. Forever grateful, I am proof of the life he saved and the love they shared.

Greater love has no one than this, that someone lay down his life for his friends.

-John 15:13

Let's Chat About It:
The Gift

1. How does my relationship with my parents reflect themes of love and strength throughout my recovery journey?
2. In what ways does the experience of receiving a kidney transplant transform me both physically and emotionally?
3. How do I navigate the delicate balance of gratitude and grief when writing a letter to my donor family? How would you approach a similar situation?
4. What role does faith play in my recovery and outlook on life after my transplant? Can you connect my experience to the Scripture mentioned in the chapter?
5. How does my decision to volunteer during my recovery, instead of rushing back to full-time work, demonstrate self-awareness and obedience?
6. How does the chapter explore the concept of "second chances"? Have you had a "second chance" moment in your life?
7. What profound "gifts" have you received in your life? How have you expressed your gratitude?
8. What are your thoughts on being a registered organ, eye, and tissue donor? What led to your position on the matter? Has this book confirmed or changed your perspective?

If something in this chapter resonated with you, I'd love to read your feedback. Please share your thoughts with an Amazon review.

13.
My Letter to Donor Families

Dear Donor Family,

There are no words that can truly express the depth of my gratitude, but I hope this letter conveys just a fraction of the appreciation I feel for the life-saving gift your loved one has given me. I want to first acknowledge the unimaginable loss you have experienced. The pain of losing someone so dear is something I cannot fully understand, but my heart goes out to you and your family. In the midst of your grief, you made an extraordinary decision—to share the gift of life through organ, eye, and tissue donation. That selfless act has given me, and many others, a second chance at life.

I now carry a part of your loved one within me. Every day, I am reminded that my life continues because of their sacrifice, and because of the compassion you demonstrated in such a difficult time. This gift has not only renewed my body but has also renewed my spirit. It has allowed me to continue the journey of life, to cherish moments with family and friends, and to pursue dreams that were once uncertain.

It is important to me that you know this: I live each day with a sense of purpose, knowing that my life is a continuation of the legacy your loved one has left behind. While my heart is full of gratitude for the second chance I've been given, I am deeply aware that this gift came from a place of loss. I carry that understanding with me every day.

Your loved one's impact reaches far beyond me. They have touched countless lives—mine, my family's, and others who received the gift of life or healing through their organ, eye, and tissue donations. I hope that, in knowing this, you find some small measure of comfort in the midst of your grief. Your loved one's spirit lives on, not only in the hearts of those who knew them, but also in those of us who have been given the chance to live because of them.

I will forever honor their memory, and I promise to live a life worthy of the gift I have been given.

With deepest gratitude and heartfelt sympathy,
Dr. Sómone D. Washington

14.
Lifelines and Collective Action

The approach to organ donation varies significantly across the globe, influencing the availability of donor organs and the effectiveness of transplantation programs. In the United States, the organ donation system is primarily opt-in, meaning individuals must actively register to become organ donors, typically through a driver's license application or dedicated donor registries. This model contrasts with opt-out systems adopted by many other countries including Spain, France, and Austria, where individuals are automatically considered organ donors unless they explicitly decline. Countries with opt-out systems generally report higher rates of organ donation. For example, Spain has one of the highest organ donation rates globally, attributed to its presumed consent law and a strong network of healthcare providers who facilitate organ recovery.

Organizations like OneLegacy play a crucial role in advocating for changes in organ donation policy, including the transition to an opt-out system in the United States. By moving to an opt-out system, the number of available organs could significantly increase. Advocates argue that many people support organ donation but have not registered due to various reasons, such as a lack of awareness on how to register and procrastination. Presumed consent would ensure that more individuals are included in the donor pool. OneLegacy often partners with lawmakers and health agencies to push for legislative changes at both state and federal levels by drafting legislation and forming coalitions.

In the United States, over 103,000 individuals are currently waiting for a life-saving organ transplant. Among them, just under 30,000 are Black/African American (U.S. Department of Health and Human Services, 2024). Despite the staggering number of deaths in the country—2,289,000 between January and September of 2023 alone (Centers for Disease Control and Prevention, 2024)—only 18,335 transplants were performed last year (UNOS, 2024). While some medical conditions prevent deceased individuals from being viable donors, a major obstacle that can be addressed is the relatively low percentage of registered organ donors. As of 2014, only about 45 percent of American adults had registered as donors (Wen, 2014).

This disparity raises an important question: why are so many Black/African Americans hesitant to register as organ donors?

To explore this issue, I conducted a small study, aiming to shed light on an area where research has been sparse, particularly over the past decade. In my investigation, I focused on the gap between the number of Black/African Americans on the transplant waitlist and the number of registered donors. I interviewed a convenience sample of six educated, middle-aged African American women in Southern California, asking ten questions to explore the factors contributing to the community's hesitation to register.

The findings from these conversations pointed to three primary concerns: a lack of education and information, deep-seated mistrust of the medical industry, and personal philosophies shaped by medical experiences. These results suggest that more targeted outreach efforts addressing these concerns could help increase donor registration within the Black/African American community.

First, the interviews revealed a significant gap in education about the organ donation process. Despite promotional efforts, conversations around organ, eye, and tissue donation are not penetrating Black/African American communities effectively. There is a noticeable absence of discussions about donation within families, across generations, and in community spaces such as churches, social organizations, and other peer groups. Without these crucial conversations, many individuals remain uninformed or misinformed about the process and its benefits.

Secondly, a profound mistrust of the medical industry looms large in the community. This mistrust has roots in a dark history of medical exploitation and abuse, including the Tuskegee Syphilis Study, where Black men were deliberately infected and denied treatment; the case of Henrietta Lacks, whose cells were used without her consent in groundbreaking medical research; and the forced sterilization of Black women. These examples are just a few in a long list of violations that have left an indelible mark on the collective memory of Black Americans. The weight of this history influences contemporary attitudes, making it critical for outreach efforts to acknowledge past wrongs while building trust in the safety and transparency of the donation process.

Lastly, personal and moral philosophies surrounding organ donation often stem from lived experiences. Whether due to personal medical challenges or witnessing the struggles of a loved one, individual experiences shape how people view organ donation. Some see it as an inherently good and charitable act, while others view it as sacrilegious or morally compromising. Those with medical education or careers in healthcare tend to be more supportive of organ donation, as their exposure to the science behind it and interactions with patients awaiting transplants provide a more direct understanding of the need. However, for many, these views remain complex and deeply personal.

The implications of these findings are clear: effective outreach efforts must be multifaceted. Initiatives should focus not only on providing accurate information but also on building trust and addressing the personal and moral concerns that shape individual decision-making. By acknowledging the historical mistrust, fostering community dialogue, and emphasizing the life-saving benefits of organ donation, it is possible to inspire more Black/African Americans to register as donors, ultimately increasing the donor pool and saving more lives.

The issues highlighted in Black/African American communities regarding organ donation—lack of education, mistrust of the medical system, and deeply rooted personal and cultural beliefs—also resonate strongly in other Brown communities, such as Latino, Indigenous, and South Asian populations. These communities face similar challenges when it comes to organ donor registration and, like Black Americans, are disproportionately represented on transplant waitlists.

To tie this information to the needs in Brown communities, we can examine parallels including the lack of education and awareness, historical and institutional mistrust, cultural and religious beliefs, health disparities, and access to medical care.

In many Brown communities, there is limited awareness and understanding of organ donation. Cultural norms around discussing death, medical procedures, and long-term health issues may prevent families from having important conversations about registering as donors. Additionally, language barriers and misinformation can further hinder access to accurate information about how organ donation works and its benefits. Outreach efforts that involve culturally competent education—delivered in multiple languages and addressing specific cultural taboos—would be critical in these communities.

For example, in Latino communities, research has shown that many people do not register as donors due to misconceptions about religion or a belief that organ donation might interfere with funeral practices, such as the desire for a body to remain intact after death. Targeted education campaigns, conducted in Spanish and led by trusted community figures like religious leaders and organizations like OneLegacy, could help alleviate these concerns.

Just as Black Americans harbor historical mistrust due to medical exploitation, many Brown communities have also faced systemic mistreatment in the healthcare system. For instance, Latino and Indigenous populations in the United States have experienced forced sterilization, limited access to healthcare, and unequal treatment in medical settings. In South Asian communities, there may be skepticism about healthcare systems in countries where corruption is perceived as rampant.

To address these concerns, outreach must include a recognition of these communities' unique histories and offer reassurances about the safeguards in place to protect donors and their families. Collaborative efforts between healthcare institutions and community leaders—such as clergy, tribal leaders, or local advocates—could help build the trust needed for people to feel confident in their decision to register as donors.

Personal and cultural beliefs regarding death, the body, and medical intervention can also contribute to low donor registration rates in Brown communities. In many cases, these beliefs are tied to religious traditions or philosophies about the sanctity of the body. For example, some in the South Asian community may believe that organ donation could hinder spiritual practices associated with death and reincarnation, or that it interferes with the soul's journey after death.

To overcome these barriers, outreach programs must respect these cultural beliefs while providing information from religious scholars or community influencers who support organ donation within the context of faith. Clarifying how organ donation aligns with the values of giving, saving lives,
and helping others could increase donor rates in communities where religious or philosophical objections play a role.

Organ donation is not just a personal choice; it's a collective responsibility that can save lives across all communities.

Brown communities often face significant health disparities, including higher rates of conditions like diabetes, high blood pressure, and chronic kidney disease, which can lead to a greater need for organ transplants. Despite this, they are less likely to register as organ donors or receive timely transplants due to systemic barriers in healthcare access and socioeconomic inequities. By focusing on how these communities are directly affected by the shortage of donors, messaging can be framed around the urgency of increasing donor registration to save lives within their own communities.

For example, outreach efforts could highlight statistics that show Latino and Indigenous Americans are more likely to experience end-stage renal disease, making the need for kidney transplants particularly urgent. Campaigns could emphasize the collective benefit of increasing donor registration within these populations to address this health crisis.

The LGBTQIA+ community faces distinct barriers when it comes to healthcare, including organ donation, many of which are rooted in historical discrimination, stigma, and a lack of tailored outreach efforts.

Much like Black and Brown communities, LGBTQIA+ individuals (many of whom are also a part of black and brown communities) often harbor mistrust of the healthcare system due to a history of discrimination. Medical policies, such as the long-standing FDA ban on blood donations from gay men, reinforce this mistrust. Many in the community may feel marginalized or excluded from discussions about healthcare, including organ donation.

It's important to reassure the LGBTQIA+ community that organ donation is inclusive and that their lives and contributions are valued. Campaigns could focus on dismantling misconceptions about their eligibility to donate and highlight the vital role that LGBTQIA+ donors play in saving lives. Partnering with LGBTQIA+ advocacy groups, healthcare providers, and influencers from the community to deliver these messages would help build trust and increase donor registrations.

LGBTQIA+ individuals (like many others) face specific health disparities, such as mental health concerns and substance use disorders, which can lead to concerns about being eligible to donate organs. Misinformation about these health conditions and their impact on donation eligibility can discourage participation.

Outreach efforts should clarify eligibility criteria and address any misunderstandings. Additionally, by spotlighting stories of LGBTQIA+ individuals who have donated or received organs, campaigns can normalize the conversation and dispel myths around eligibility.

The LGBTQIA+ community is often rooted in mutual care and support. Framing organ donation as a continuation of this ethic—saving lives and helping others—could resonate deeply. Highlighting how organ donation can be a powerful way to give back to the community, regardless of one's gender identity or sexual orientation, may encourage more people to register as donors.

While Caucasian Americans are the majority of registered organ donors, there are still many who do not participate due to a combination of complacency, misinformation, and personal or philosophical beliefs.

In the Caucasian community, where registration rates are often higher than in minority communities, some individuals may not feel the same urgency to register because they believe enough people are already participating. Additionally, misconceptions about the medical process or the belief that organ donation is something they'll address later in life can lead to inaction.

Campaigns aimed at the Caucasian community should focus on breaking the complacency by sharing stories that highlight the ongoing, critical shortage of organs. They can also emphasize that registering is an act of solidarity and responsibility for the broader community. Messaging could include real-life examples of how quickly circumstances can change, showing that anyone could find themselves in need of an organ transplant unexpectedly.

Like other communities, Caucasians may harbor misconceptions about organ donation. Some fear that signing up as a donor might lead to inadequate medical care in an emergency or believe that certain health conditions make them ineligible to donate.

Education campaigns should focus on debunking myths about organ donation, including the fact that registering as a donor does not affect the level of care people receive in life-threatening situations. By promoting positive stories from healthcare professionals and individuals who have benefited from organ donation, these campaigns can provide reassurance and clarity.

Some Caucasians may avoid registering due to personal or religious beliefs about bodily integrity after death or concerns about the morality of organ donation.

These concerns, while not unique to Caucasians, can be more prevalent in certain subsets of this community.

Tailored outreach should address these concerns by involving religious leaders and philosophers who can provide ethical and theological perspectives on organ donation. Many religious organizations support organ donation as a charitable act, and highlighting this in community-specific campaigns could help ease apprehensions.

At the heart of organ donation lies a universal truth: regardless of race, ethnicity, gender identity, sexual orientation, medical status, or age, we all have the power to save lives. While each community faces unique challenges when it comes to organ donation, we are united by the shared potential to make a great difference. Whether it's overcoming historic mistrust, addressing misinformation, or fostering a sense of urgency, the key to increasing donor registration is creating a space where every community feels informed, supported, and empowered to act.

The organ transplant waitlist transcends boundaries, affecting people from all walks of life. By working together, we can ensure that organ donation becomes a common conversation in every household, every community center, and every place of worship. Through collaboration, education, and a commitment to breaking down barriers, we can create a culture where organ donation is seen not only as a personal choice but as an act of solidarity that saves lives across all communities.

When we address the specific needs of each group while embracing our shared humanity, we make organ donation more inclusive, equitable, and impactful. Ultimately, the future of organ donation rests in our ability to come together as one, to raise awareness, and to recognize that the act of giving life knows no boundaries. With more registered donors from all communities, we can ensure that every person in need has a fighting chance, and that hope is available to all.

And do not forget to do good and to share with others, for with such sacrifices God is pleased.

-Hebrews 13:16

Let's Chat About It: Lifelines and Collective Action

1. What personal experiences or beliefs shape your perspective on organ donation?
2. How do cultural attitudes toward organ donation differ among the communities discussed (Black, Brown, LGBTQIA+, and Caucasian)? What can be done to address these differences?
3. What are your thoughts on the opt-in vs. opt-out organ donation systems? Which system do you believe would be more effective in increasing donor registrations, and why?
4. How can education and awareness campaigns be tailored to engage different communities effectively? What role do you think personal stories play in this?
5. Why is building trust in the healthcare system particularly important for marginalized communities regarding organ donation? How can healthcare providers work to rebuild this trust?
6. What are some ways that you can contribute to this awareness campaign within your circle of influence?
7. What important points to consider have been left out of this chapter or is typically missed in conversations around organ, eye, and tissue donation?

Did a part of this chapter stand out to you? I'd love to know your thoughts—feel free to leave a review on Amazon.

Epilogue
Living Testimony

At the writing of this book, thirteen years have passed since the pivotal moment that I received a second chance at life through kidney transplant. As I reflect on the life I've been privileged to live since then, I'm filled with gratitude. My journey has taken me to California, where I've embraced a vibrant life. Along the way, I've explored various facets of my career—from working as a software analyst to founding my own tech education company. I've found joy and purpose in public speaking, coaching, consulting, and now proudly garnering the title of published author.

My academic pursuits have also flourished; I've earned a second master's degree and been awarded an honorary doctorate in humanities. Yet, the most cherished moments have been spent creating lasting memories with my parents, extended family, and friends. These connections are the true treasures of my life.

Words often fall short in expressing gratitude for a gift as profound as life itself. In recognition of this, I've served as a OneLegacy Ambassador for almost ten years, dedicating my time to raise awareness about the vital importance of registering as an organ, eye, and tissue donor. Sharing my story is my way of contributing to this cause and offering a tangible "thank you" to my donor family.

As I look ahead, I eagerly anticipate meeting the love of my life, continuing my adventures across the globe, and settling into a fulfilling existence. I reflect on the myriads of experiences I've had—the highs and lows, the triumphs and missteps, even living through the challenges of a global pandemic. Each moment has been a blessing, and I'm extremely thankful for the opportunity to still be here, savoring it all.

I stand humbled, recognizing that my life has been chosen as a testament to God's love. This journey is not just mine; it's a shared tapestry of faith, hope, resilience, and the enduring power of human connection… the best of all things.

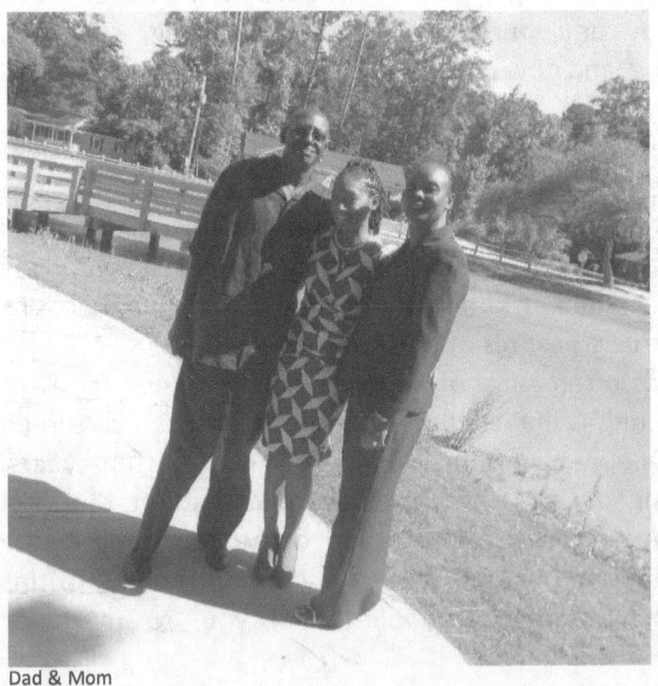

Dad & Mom

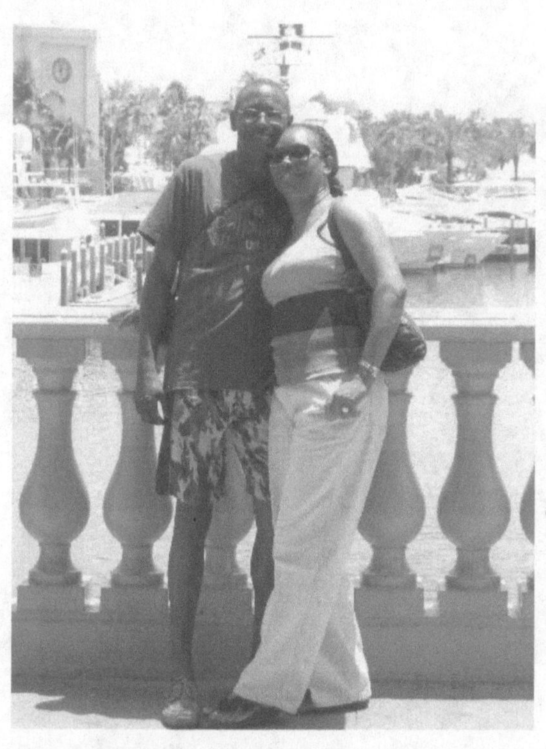

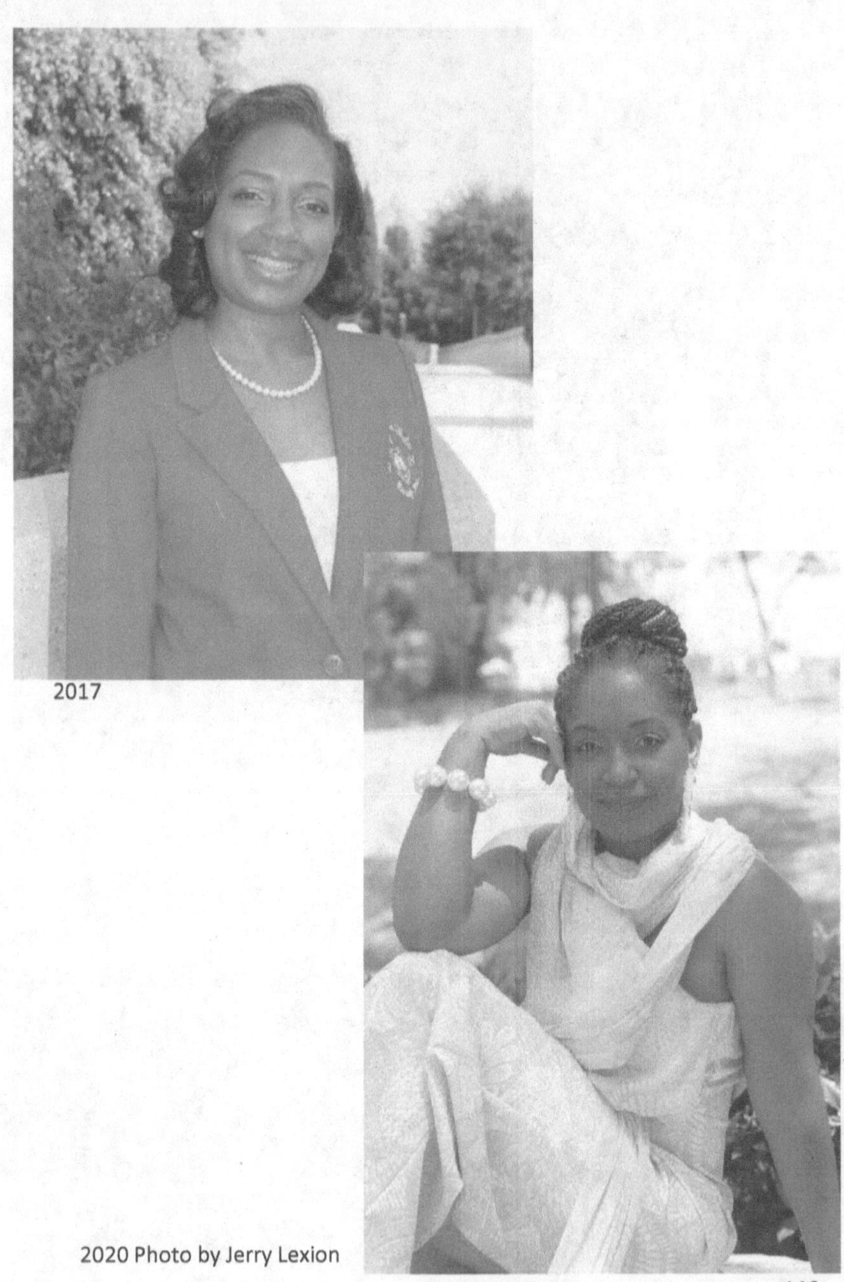

2017

2020 Photo by Jerry Lexion

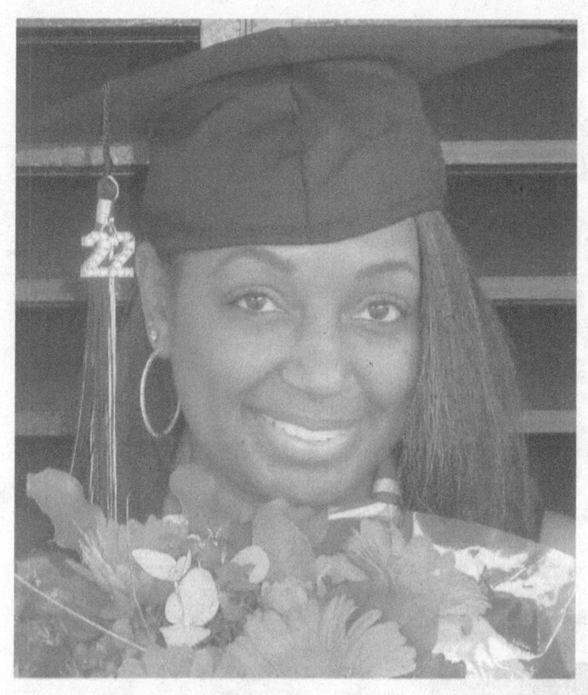

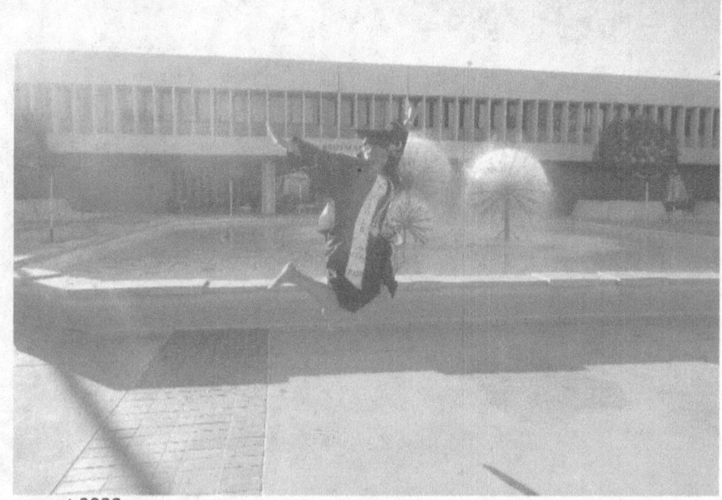

Commencement 2022

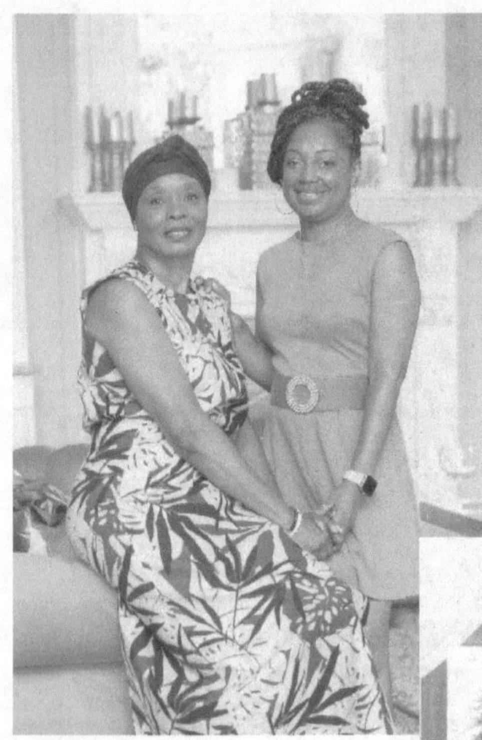

Mom and I

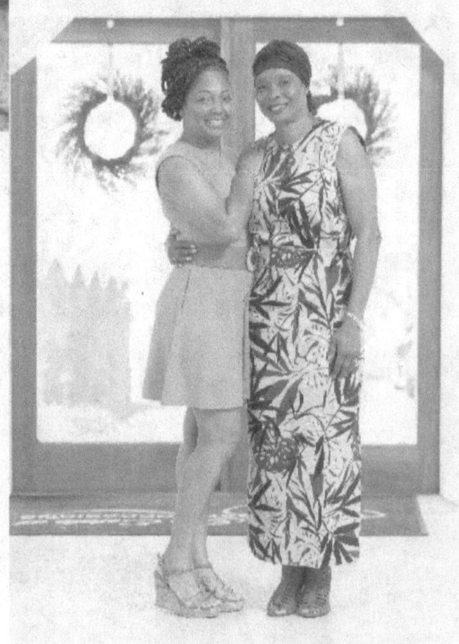

Mom's Surprise Birthday Party 2024

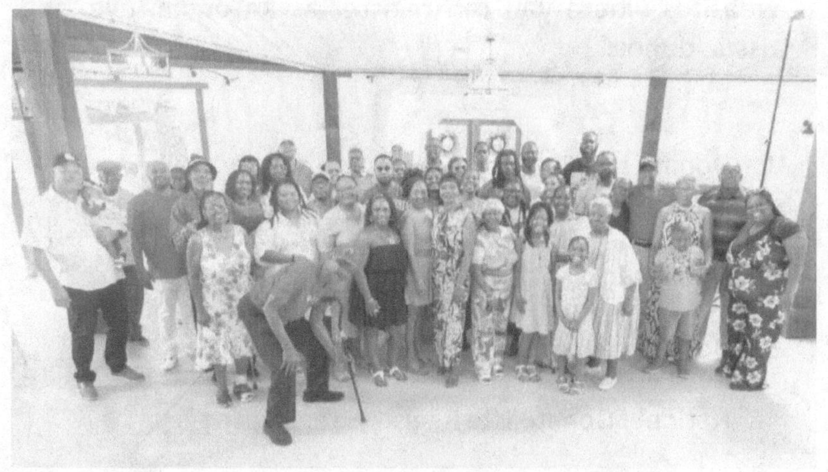

Are you ready to leave a lasting legacy? Here's a list of ten websites where you can register as an organ, eye, and tissue donor:

1. Donate Life California – Somone's Story: https://register.donatelifecalifornia.org/somonesstory
2. OneLegacy: https://www.onelegacy.org/wp/
3. Donate Life America: donatelife.net
4. National Donate Life Registry: registerme.org
5. American Transplant Foundation: americantransplantfoundation.org
6. United Network for Organ Sharing (UNOS): unos.org
7. National Kidney Foundation: kidney.org
8. Department of Motor Vehicles: https://www.dmv.org/organ-donor.php
9. New England Donor Services: nedonate.org
10. Lifesharers: lifesharers.org

These sites provide information on how to register, as well as details about the donation process and its significance.

I stand humbled, recognizing that my life has been chosen as a testament to God's love.

Finally, brothers and sisters, whatever is true,
whatever is noble, whatever is right, whatever
is pure, whatever is lovely, whatever is
admirable—if anything is excellent or
praiseworthy—think about such things.

-Philippians 4:8

Let's Chat About It:

Living Testimony

1. How has my journey shaped my perspective on gratitude? Can you relate to any moments in your life where gratitude shifted your outlook?
2. I mention moving to California and starting anew. What are some significant transitions you've experienced, and how did they impact your personal growth?
3. How do I express my faith throughout my journey? In what ways do you think faith can influence resilience and personal development?
4. The epilogue highlights creating memories with family and friends. How do relationships shape our experiences and help us navigate challenges?
5. I have become a OneLegacy Ambassador to promote organ donation awareness. What role do you think personal stories play in advocacy efforts?
6. How do our experiences during the global pandemic reflect broader themes of resilience? What lessons can we learn from such experiences?
7. What are your final thoughts after reading this book?
8. Who in your life could benefit from reading this book? Why?

If this chapter left an impression on you, I'd be so grateful if you shared your thoughts by leaving a review on Amazon.

References

American Heart Association. Health Threats from High Blood Pressure (https://www.heart.org/en/health-topics/high-blood-pressure/health-threats-from-high-blood-pressure).

Centers for Disease Control and Prevention. (2024, January 19). *National Vital Statistics System: State and National Provisional Counts*. National Center for Health Statistics, CDC. (https://www.cdc.gov/nchs/nvss/vsrr/provisional-tables.htm).

Cleveland Clinic. (2021, August 18). *Dialysis: Types, how it works, Procedure & Side effects*. Cleveland Clinic. (https://my.clevelandclinic.org/health/treatments/14618-dialysis).

Guerra, G. [Giselle]. (2011, January 20). *Follow-up Transplant Clinic Note*. Miami, FL: Jackson Memorial Hospital.

Mayo Foundation for Medical Education and Research. (2023, February 9). *Creatinine Test*. Mayo Clinic. (https://www.mayoclinic.org/tests-procedures/creatinine-test/about/pac-20384646#:~:text=A%20creatinine%20test%20is%20a,a%20waste%20product%20in%20urine). Accessed 5/14/2024.

Merriam-Webster. (2024). *Hedonism definition & meaning*. Merriam-Webster. https://www.merriam-webster.com/dictionary/hedonism#:~:text=%3A%20the%20doctrine%20that%20pleasure%20or,of%20selfish%20hedonism%20Donald%20Armstrong

Staff, Y. (2024). *1 Thessalonians 5:16-18 Rejoice always, pray continually, give thanks in all circumstances; for this is God's will for you in Christ Jesus.: New International Version (NIV):* YouVersion | The Bible App | Bible.com. https://www.bible.com/bible/111/1TH.5.NIV

Staff, Y. (2024). *Philippians 4:12 I know what it is to be in need, and I know what it is to have plenty. I have learned the secret of being content in any and every situation, whether well fed or hungry, whether living in plenty or in: New International Version (NIV):* YouVersion | The Bible App | Bible.com. https://www.bible.com/bible/111/PHP.4.12.NIV

United Network for Organ Sharing (UNOS). (2021, January 17). *Transplant Trends: OPTN Metrics.* Organ Procurement and Transplantation Network (OPTN). https://insights.unos.org/OPTN-metrics/

United Network for Organ Sharing, UNOS. (2022). *Records: Adult Kidney Transplant Recipient Registration*

(Report No. 0915-0157). United Network for Organ Sharing.

U.S. Department of Health and Human Services. (2024, May 27). Organ Procurement and Transplantation Network: National Data. https://optn.transplant.hrsa.gov/data/view-data-reports/national-data/#

Washington, Somone (2021). *Doesn't Everyone Want to be a Hero? A Qualitative Ethnographic Study of Apprehensions Among Black/African Americans Surrounding Organ, Eye, and Tissue Donation Registry.* https://somonewashington0.wixsite.com/eportfolio/post/student-learning-outcome-4

Wen, T. (2014, November 10). *Why Don't More People Want to Donate Their Organs?* The Atlantic Monthly Group. https://www.theatlantic.com/health/archive/2014/11/why-dont-people-want-to-donate-their-organs/382297/

Post-Credits Scene

In an early chapter of this book titled "A Journey to Jamaica," I invited you to accompany me on a transformative mission trip that reshaped my understanding of purpose and community. As I prepared for this life-changing journey, a powerful prophecy from a woman bishop struck a deep chord within me. She proclaimed that I was destined to be “an Esther for my people”—a call that carried both immense weight and a touch of confusion.

You might be curious as to why I chose to share this prophecy with you and how it weaves into the larger tapestry of my life’s narrative. The true depth of this prophecy will be revealed in my next book, ***My Name is Esther***. You may think you know, but trust me, you have no idea. Will you join me once more on this journey I call life?

Acknowledgements

A special thank you to the major contributors that helped make this work a reality.

Dr. Catrena Eliott – my book coach
https://www.drcatrenaelliott.com/

Susan Jacobs – editor of the article that ignited a flame
https://www.csulb.edu/news/article/csulb-staffer-reflects-gratitude-after-life-saving-organ-transplant

Dr. Valerie Rhoden – my mentor and author of *Leading from the Inside Out: Wisdom for Compassionate Leaders* *https://www.amazon.com/-/he/Dr-Valmarie-Ward-Rhoden/dp/0578832089*

Dennard Mitchell – my book writing consultant and author of *Write. Publish. Leverage.*
https://dennardmitchell.com/

OneLegacy – providing a space for me to pay it forward and hone my storytelling skills
https://www.onelegacy.org/wp/ambassadors

Family – encouragement and support

Friends – everyone who offered advice on book titles and book cover designs: *Susan Fowler, Jacqueline Jones, Miesha McClendon, Garrett Robinson, Dr. Gwendolyn Bryant, Sheila Wiley, Tasha Carouthers, Dr. Gardenia Bulluck, Kissy Talley, Chereise Martin, KayCee*

About the Author

Dr. Sómone D. Washington is an accomplished Learning and Development professional with over 20 years of experience designing impactful educational experiences. She is the founder and owner of Kiasi Technology Solutions, where she leverages her expertise to create innovative learning solutions. Dr. Washington's academic achievements include degrees from Florida International University, Barry University, and California State University, Long Beach, along with an honorary Doctor of Humanity.

A dedicated member of Delta Sigma Theta Sorority, Inc. for nearly 25 years, Dr. Washington has consistently demonstrated her commitment to leadership, service, community, and social action. She has passionately shared her story to raise awareness about the critical need for organ, eye, and tissue donors, especially within Black and brown communities.

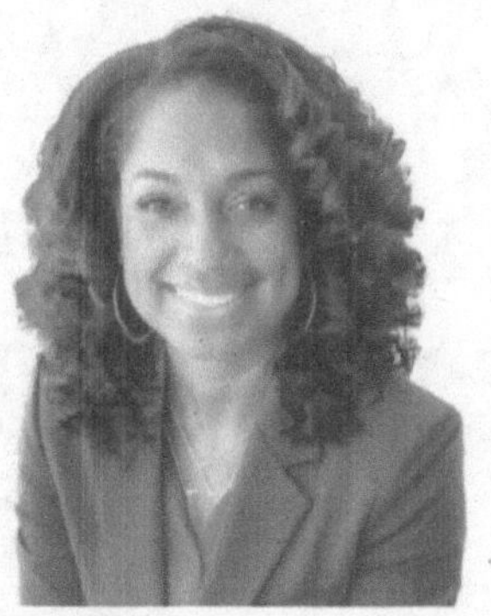

Dr. Washington's dedication to this cause extends to her work as an ambassador for OneLegacy, a leading organization focused on public education and family support for organ donation. Through speaking engagements and collaborations with medical professionals, she inspires others to consider becoming donors, emphasizing the disproportionate need for transplants within minority populations.

In her professional life, Dr. Washington continues to excel as a public speaker, author, business strategist and coach, book development consultant, technology learning facilitator, digital implementation professional, and an award-winning software analyst at a university in Southern California, where she resides. Her inspiring story, professional accomplishments, and ongoing advocacy work reflect her unwavering commitment to making a positive difference in the world.

www.ingramcontent.com/pod-product-compliance
Lightning Source LLC
LaVergne TN
LVHW031316150826
845672LV00010B/2803

* 9 7 9 8 2 1 8 4 9 9 9 1 4 *